MIDWIFERY OF THE SOUL:
A HOLISTIC PERSPECTIVE ON PSYCHOANALYSIS

MIDWIFERY OF THE SOUL:

A HOLISTIC PERSPECTIVE ON PSYCHOANALYSIS

Collected Papers of
Margaret Arden

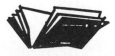

FREE ASSOCIATION BOOKS / LONDON / NEW YORK

Published in 1998 by
Free Association Books Ltd
57 Warren Street, London W1P 5PA
and 70 Washington Square South,
New York, NY 10012–1091

ISBN 1 85343 389 6 hardback; 1 85343 391 8 paperback

A CIP catalogue record for this book is available from
the British Library.

Produced for Free Association Books Ltd by
Chase Production Services, Chadlington, OX7 3LN
Printed in the EC by J.W. Arrowsmith Ltd, Bristol

For Michael

Ever splitting the light!
How often do they strive to divide
that which, despite everything, would always
remain single and whole.
Goethe

Contents

Acknowledgements

My special thanks to Paul Williams for believing in this book sufficiently to commission the last chapter, and for his assistance in making its publication a reality.

I would like to thank Elizabeth Spillius for her positive criticism, and Linda Holt for her sustained encouragement. Jill Duncan has been providing me with library services since I first began to write, and I cannot imagine doing without her help and support. The friends and colleagues who have read my manuscripts over the years are too numerous to name, but they all contributed to the final result.

Foreword

Elizabeth Spillius

I first met Margaret Arden forty years ago when I was doing an anthropological study of a mental hospital, a hospital which in her Introduction to the present book she describes, elegantly and accurately, as 'a benign patriarchal system of obedience and delegated responsibility [in which] the staff had security of tenure, and the patients a protected environment where they were allowed to be mad.' Soon the hospital suffered the benefits of 'science' – drugs, new research, an anti-institutionalisation campaign, reorganisation – all with the best intent, but slowly the safe place to be mad and to learn about madness was transformed and destroyed. Perhaps this was one of the several experiences which contributed to Margaret's dislike of science as a narrow cause-and-effect world view.

The things I remember about Margaret then are the same qualities that strike one now: a profound respect for truth as she sees it, integrity, ability to think for herself without having to follow accepted views. And so in this book we find her recognising explicitly that the ideas came into her mind – uninvited, as she says – in psychoanalytic sessions were not the 'scientific' content of psychoanalytic theory but the ideas of the Christianity she had been immersed in at school. It was those ideas that led her to rediscover a sense of wholeness in the healing process, in patients, and, potentially, in psychoanalytic theory.

Although she does not quite say so directly except to some extent in 'Freud and Jung', I think that Margaret was and is deeply impressed by Freud's basic conception: the idea of the unconscious and especially of its having its own peculiar non-rational logic, the primary process, revealed to Freud through the analysis of dreams. What she is not impressed by is the idea that this primary process must be modified into or at the very least controlled by the secondary process, the logic of common sense. Although Margaret does not describe in detail the aspects of Freud's thought that follow the tenets of the materialistic cause-and-effect science of the nineteenth century, I believe it is her belief that the basic difficulty with Freud's science is that its aim is to subject the primary process to the logic of the secondary process. She feels this aim does not do justice to the primary process, without which there can be no imagination, no creativity, none of the cultural accomplishments of human societies. She wants a theory in which integration rather than control is the motif. Hence her desire for a holistic approach.

In search for understanding of a holistic world view Margaret has gone to psychoanalysts but far beyond as well: to Marjorie Brierley, Sylvia Payne and Charles Rycroft; to Matte Blanco's idea of bi-logic; to Bateson's ideas of double binds and the unity of mind and evolution; to David Bohm's idea of the holomovement and the implicate order; to Rupert Sheldrake's theory of 'morphic resonance'; to Gleick's chaos theory; to Lovelock's Gaia hypothesis; to Arieti's idea of tertiary mental process; to Goethe's science. All of these ideas she expounds with exemplary clarity.

I find an occasional ambiguity in Margaret's exposition of holistic theory. Is the aim to integrate primary and secondary process, femininity and masculinity, implicate and explicate orders? Or is one of these logics the ultimate reality of which the other is or should be a part, a perspective? Thus, for example, in describing Bohm's theory of the holomovement and the implicate order she says that 'holomovement [the ultimate, unknowable reality] is the primary process and the unique human achievement is the ability to extract useful explicate order reality from the holomovement in the form of secondary process logical thinking' (p. 42). But she also speaks of Arieti's idea (1976) that creativity requires *combination* of primary and secondary process. 'The new order', Margaret says, 'can be grasped imaginatively by people who can combine primary and secondary process thinking ... what is required is a shift into a higher logical type of thinking as Bateson described', (p. 41). In this case the 'higher logical type of thinking' is not primary process; it is an *integration* of primary and secondary process thinking.

Similarly in 'A concept of femininity: Sylvia Payne's 1935 paper reassessed' (Chapter 3), Margaret states, in line with Brierley and Payne, that femininity is in itself an integrating force. But she also suggests 'that the primary process is feminine and secondary process is masculine thinking' (p. 48) – an idea that has not been further explored, so far as I know. In keeping with this differention she says that 'the male and female [are] complementary opposites which need to be integrated for healthy living'.

Perhaps it is my nineteenth-century cause-and-effect 'scientific' attitude that leads me to make this distinction between, on the one hand, a model in which primary process is basic and secondary process is derivative, and, on the other hand, a model in which primary and secondary processes are equal but different and need to be integrated to form a new and higher synthesis. Perhaps the important point is that primary process should be given its due.

Many readers are likely to share my difficulty in understanding the way Margaret is using the diverse theories she discusses. They will be tempted to try to find a single message that they can take from the book, which is not what Margaret intends the reader to do. She is, on the contrary, inviting the reader to follow her on her journey, looking at the views of various authors who are trying to explain how the universe and the mind, which is part of the universe, work, and seeing psychoanalysis as a microcosm where they can be further explored. Such an exploration should broaden one's vision, promoting integration rather than fragmentation. And, as she puts it, the psychoanalyst acts as midwife – hence the title of her book – 'assisting the patient to find his or her truth in a self-authenticating way.'

To my way of thinking, however, Margaret is too modest, too much inclined to express her ideas through outlining the ideas of others. She describes what is wrong with cause-and-effect science, including that of Freud, and, through the medium of exploring the ideas of recent and more enlightened scientists – but including the science of Goethe too – she gives a general characterisation of the sort of holistic theory that would be more appropriate for psychoanalysis. But I believe that much work remains to be done in developing a clinical theory that would do proper justice to her sense of therapeutic truth. She gives enticing glimpses of her way of working with patients which illustrate her sensitive capacity to understand and help them, but these movements towards wholeness are not linked with the overall holistic approach in a way that would show how we might move towards a specifically psychoanalytic holistic theory.

So her book is tantalising, giving one a vivid awareness of her sense of personal and clinical truth, but leaving one hoping that the shape of an appropriate holistic psychoanalytic theory will emerge in the future. In the meantime her thoughtful and unconventional book will inspire readers to think about the problem, each in his own way.

Introduction

This book records the intellectual journey made by one psycho-analyst between 1980 and 1997. The papers are printed in chronological order with only minor editorial changes. It has not been possible to adapt the early chapters in the light of later knowledge; they have to stand as they were originally conceived. The ideas which are discussed in the early papers recur throughout and are present in the final chapter, the connecting theme being the concept of wholeness.

I began my career as a psychoanalyst by accepting the Freudian teaching I had absorbed (perhaps too early in life) during my training, not questioning the idea that psychoanalysis was a science. As I tried to reconcile what I had been taught with my own point of view, I had to go back to basics and learn about the history of ideas. On reflection, I think that just as important as my pursuit of truth was my willingness to admit what I did not know. This is not so much a virtue as an incapacity for identifying completely with any one school of thought.

I had studied science at school and went straight from school to medical school, where the first two pre-clinical years were devoted to learning more science. At that time the practice of medicine was still an art as well as a science, and on the wards students were made aware of their lack of two skills: we were no good at examining patients and we lacked an appropriate bedside manner. It was the discrepancy between the ideal of kindliness and respect and the actual behaviour of consultants to patients that determined my move into psychiatry as soon as I had completed my pre-registration year. Looking back I can see that patients were often put in a double bind; on the surface they were treated with courtesy but there was an unspoken requirement to submit to the power of the consultant.

Old-fashioned mental hospitals are outwardly grim, but in 1954 psychotropic drugs had not arrived, and the hospital was run by the Medical Superintendent who held ultimate power. Within a benign patriarchal system of obedience and delegated responsibility the staff had security of tenure, and the patients a protected environment where they were allowed to be mad. Eccentric behaviour was tolerated from both patients and staff, and it was not only the patients who became institutionalised. Fortunately for me I arrived by chance at a hospital where many of the junior doctors were travelling to London daily to undertake psychoanalytic training. I was welcomed and appreciated, and I found I had a natural bent for psychotherapy. I learned a great deal of psychiatry while I trained as an analyst, which has stood me in good stead.

It was not until I started working as a psychoanalyst in private practice many years later that I became fascinated by the problem of the gap between psychoanalytic theory and practice. Like many trainees, I was young and impressionable, with an idealised notion of how I should think and talk to my patients. Having to rely on my own judgement in sessions made me realise that my experience bore little relation to my mental picture of Freud's theories and his way of working. I was forced to realise that the only thing I could rely on was my sense of the truth of what was going on in the consulting room.

At that time, the late 1970s, it was still customary for anyone presenting a paper at a Scientific Meeting of the British Psychoanalytical Society to make references to Freud and connections between their own ideas and Freud's. In this way the body of knowledge that was psychoanalysis was preserved and extended. There was no means of challenging anything outmoded or wrong. Several authors had already questioned Freud's theoretical views but analysts in general were living with the state of affairs I have described, and were tying themselves in mental knots in order to think for themselves.

When I began private practice I was still under the influence of the idea that psychoanalysis was a science. I had a guilty feeling that there was something wrong with following my own instincts rather than applying what I had been taught. I found myself asking, about each patient I saw, what their life was about; and this mirrored many of my questions about myself. Part of my attitude was the result of an unexamined acceptance of my parents' naive atheism, because it agreed with Freud's views on religion. Examining my reactions to my patients forced me to make a discovery which took me by surprise. I realised that my values were not based on my parents' views, nor on the psychoanalysis that I had been taught. What came into my mind uninvited, time and again, was the Christianity in which I had been immersed at school. For a long time this was implicit rather than explicit in my papers, but one aspect of my journey has been the reconciliation of science and religion.

It took me many years to understand the significance in our culture of Cartesian dualism. As the result of the separation of subject and object, of thinking and feeling, there has been a progressive alienation from a sense of wholeness, which is now taken as absolute by many people. A scientific view of the world is mistakenly thought to be a description of how the world really is; it is not recognised that scientific concepts use words and mathematical symbols to describe a simulacrum of the phenomenal world. We cannot achieve an objective view of a world of which we are inescapably a part. Psychoanalysis is recognised as a path to the rediscovery of a sense of wholeness. However, the means by which this happens is largely absent from psychoanalytic theory.

I was discovering the significance of Cartesian dualism at the same time as I was learning about the theories which contradicted it. In particular, quantum theory shows how rational knowledge gives us information only about how our instruments work, whether they are sense organs or sophisticated scientific equipment. Scientists have repeatedly claimed to be approaching some kind of ultimate reality, which subsequently proves unattainable.

After twenty years I can be more explicit about the religious issue. I believe there is such a thing as psychic truth, which can be found in all religions as well as in psychoanalysis. This is an elusive concept, and religions are just as subject to distortion and misuse as any other theory. An analyst working with the right kind of attention will have little doubt about what the truth is when it appears. The patient needs the analyst to recognise the truth of who he or she is. The work of the transference and countertransference enables the truth to be made manifest in the consulting room. The analyst acts as midwife, assisting the patient to find his or her truth, in a self-authenticating way.

This preoccupation has given me the advantage of being able to think about good and evil without having to justify it. I am a Christian in the sense that Christianity means a great deal to me and it is the only religion of which I have personal knowledge. While I accept the values of Christianity, I do not feel bound by its creed. I have felt at home in the Independent Group of psychoanalysts because of the unspoken tradition, dating from pre-war days, in which English analysts were part of a society in which Christian values were taken for granted. I acknowledge a debt to the work of Marjorie Brierley, Sylvia Payne, John Rickman, Donald Winnicott, Marion Milner and Charles Rycroft. I feel part of a tradition within psychoanalysis which is more concerned with symbolic meanings than with scientific procedure. In my idiosyncratic version, this way of working is consistent with Christian spirituality. For me the transformation produced by insight in the consulting room is symbolically equivalent to the spiritual journey towards enlightenment. Psychoanalysis is a new version of the ancient theme shared by all the great religions. The loss of illusion, the giving up of attachment to a false reality, the inevitability of suffering and expiation are all present in psychoanalysis. The sea of faith may have withdrawn but the need for belief systems remains. Many of the theories which are now fashionable only make sense to those who are stranded on the naked shingles unable to remember what faith was.

Psychoanalysts talk about good and bad internal objects; Christians about love and hate. I think in terms of interactions between people which are either loving or hating, fragmenting or connecting. I see this as a form of ultimate knowledge, and every person who seeks analysis is on a personal pilgrimage. It is the language of the individual that we must use and from which we must shape our responses. It is only at one remove that we have mental furniture in the form of theories which support our thinking. I am as antipathetic to psychoanalytic theories which impose conventions on the patient as I am to fundamentalist Christian manipulation of the faithful.

Another basic Christian idea which is important to me as an analyst is that Jesus said, 'Unless you become like little children, you shall not enter the kingdom of heaven.' This is my marker of the true self. False self behaviour is usually manipulative and destructive of psychic truth. All our theories can be seen as ways of unravelling the destructive processes or defences which the patient uses. The miracle of psychoanalysis – and it is a miracle – is that when a person comes to understand the core of his or her childhood experience, all the anger, all the rejection of life, turns out to have been for one purpose – to preserve, at whatever cost, the child who is capable of love.

Each of my papers has been inspired by reading a particular author. Gregory Bateson was the first to engage me in my search for alternative theories. *Steps to an Ecology of Mind* (Bateson 1973) provided me with a way of conceptualising my questions. Bateson wrote: 'The individual mind is immanent but not only in the body. It is immanent also in pathways and messages outside the body; and there is a larger Mind of which the individual mind is only a sub-system.' I found it liberating to be able to go beyond the limitations of the individual patient's repetition of the past in the relationship to me.

Eric Rayner's (1981) paper on infinite experiences introduced me to Matte Blanco and his theory of bi-logic. I was hooked into this difficult but fascinating subject not by the intensity of Matte Blanco's writing, but by his frontispiece of a Byzantine mosaic of an archangel. A seventeen-line caption discusses the multidimensionality of the archangel's wings. Matte Blanco suggests that the artist intuitively conceived the archangel as governed by laws which are beyond those of Aristotelian logic, but which could be translated or unfolded into those laws. This is a striking use of logic to connect with the unitary view of the pre-Renaissance, pre-perspective mind. Matte Blanco achieved his insights through many years of studying schizophrenic patients' use of words.

It now seems presumptuous of me to have written about two such diverse authors in my first published paper. There is an obvious interpretation that by arranging a marriage between two sets of ideas I overcame my anxiety about expressing my own views in print.

David Bohm I discovered by chance, or synchronicity; my eye was caught by the photograph on the cover of *Wholeness and the Implicate Order* as I walked through a bookshop. When I first read it, I had little understanding of the way in which his holistic theory resonates with many religious writings of the past, but I intuitively connected the unfolding function with Matte Blanco.

My paper on femininity (Chapter 3) was written when I became aware that very few analysts had heard of Sylvia Payne's 1935 paper, 'A Concept of Femininity', let alone read it. There was a good reason for this: it was published in the *British Journal of Medical Psychology*. At that time Freud's papers on female sexuality were only recently published and the nature of femininity was still being explored. Ernest Jones was the founder-editor of the *International Journal of Psychoanalysis*, and there were diplomatic reasons for Sylvia Payne's choice of journal. The emphasis in my paper is on the integrating function of feminine experience as one aspect of the holistic ideas I was exploring.

The next paper, 'The Pattern which Connects' (Chapter 4) had been developing at the same time. I reviewed the second edition of Rupert Sheldrake's book *A New Science of Life* and unwittingly perpetuated an error of omission in that book, which must be explained. By using the term 'morphic resonance' for the unknown factor in his theory of formative causation, Sheldrake assumes and bypasses the whole field of morphogenesis. Knowledge of the processes of morphogenesis in plants and animals has increased enormously since 1985, both as a result of experimental work and also through modelling of these processes with computers. The limitations of neo-Darwinist theory have been revealed by the demonstration of the patterns that arise spontaneously in living and inanimate matter. Understanding of morphogenesis has been transformed by the discovery that similar types of dynamic behaviour can arise from complex systems irrespective of their material composition. Brian Goodwin summarises the change that has taken place:

Instead of the opposition of physics and biology, the former as the science of rational order deduced from fixed laws of nature and the latter described (since Darwin) as a historical science, physics is becoming more historical and generative while biology becomes more exact and rational. (Goodwin 1994: 191)

In other words, the reductionist aspect of neo-Darwinism, which produced the gene as the unit of survival, has been superseded. Instead biologists are once again concerned with the functions of organisms, singly and in groups, and the spontaneous emergence of life processes in which co-operation is just as important as competition.

The paper 'Freud and Jung' (Chapter 5) continues further in the same direction. I find the idea of the collective unconscious a useful way of expressing the innate capacities of the mind. Archetypal patterns of behaviour also seem to me to have a basic biological significance, even if there is not yet a satisfactory way of accounting for them. I wrote the paper long before Richard Noll's book *The Jung Cult* (1994) shed new light on the intellectual climate of the early years of the twentieth century. In particular, Noll suggests that the Mithraic myth of the solar wind was common knowledge, falsifying Jung's use of his patient's fantasy to demonstrate the existence of the collective unconscious. Re-reading my paper in the light of Noll's book, I decided not to change it. To do so would be to adopt a narrow academic viewpoint which is the opposite of my intentions. Noll has shown that many of the ideas current at the turn of the century were not academically respectable. Discrediting famous people who were once idealised has become an industry, but ideas cannot be judged by the behaviour of their originators. There are many examples of Jung's creative use of dreams and imagination which enrich the Freudian view of dreams. This is discussed further in Chapter 7. The interconnected themes of archetypal images in dreams, unconscious communication, prophetic dreams and thought transference run through the book. I have watched with interest as these subjects have gradually become respectable as hard evidence accumulates.

The last paper, 'Dreams, Imagination and the Self' (Chapter 8), closes the circle with my thoughts about Goethe. I was following up Owen Barfield's suggestion, made many years ago, that it was time for Goethe's scientific ideas to be re-examined (Barfield 1988). Barfield was a significant influence in my coming to understand the role of perception in the creation of false images, which in our materialistic culture are mistaken for the true reality. Since I wrote that paper, I have found my view of Goethe's significance already stated by two very different authors: Milan Kundera writing in 1990, and the composer Victor Ullman who wrote about Goethe while imprisoned in Theresienstadt in 1944. Interest in Goethe's science is now growing and several books have been published on his relevance for the new developments in scientific thought (Goodwin 1994: 122–3).

These papers were written over a period of fifteen years, using the conventional terminology of collective nouns in which 'his' should be read as implying 'his or her'. Similarly, 'man' signifies humankind. In Chapter 8 this convention has been maintained for the sake of continuity of style, and does not imply neglect of gender issues.

1 Infinite Sets and Double Binds[*]

It is impossible to open a psychoanalytical journal without finding at least one paper which deals with the problem of bringing theory up to date. There are widely differing approaches, but many authors seem to be asking the same question: How can we reconcile the essential truth of Freud's discoveries with the advances in other disciplines which make his work seem so out of date?

The requirement which has not been met is for a way of expressing psychoanalytical ideas in a form which is compatible with ideas from other sources, and which can incorporate such ideas into a specifically psychoanalytical language. I propose to discuss the work of Gregory Bateson and Ignacio Matte Blanco, two very different thinkers, in the hope of showing that they have ideas in common. My thesis is that by bringing together the ideas of these two authors the theory of neurotic conflict can be reformulated without damage to Freud's original meaning.

I shall give a brief account of the ideas I have developed from my reading of Bateson (1973) and Matte Blanco (1975) and then give clinical examples of how these ideas can be used in analysis. I shall begin with an account of Russell's theory of logical types, which is used by both authors. I am indebted to Eric Rayner's paper on Matte Blanco (Rayner 1981), without which I would not even have begun to read *The Unconscious as Infinite Sets*. Russell's theory of logical types states that there is a discontinuity between a class and its members so that a member cannot represent the class. The reason a member of a class of objects or ideas cannot represent that class is because it

---

[*] First published in the *International Journal of Psychoanalysis*, 1984, 65: 443–52.

belongs to a different logical category. An apple is a fruit, but it does not possess all the characteristics of fruit. In the subset of apples any apple can stand for all apples, and any pear can stand for all pears in the subset of pears; but if one wants to denote the two subsets together, then the category of fruit is required to encompass both.

Bateson uses this concept of logical typing to describe human relationships. The signals exchanged between people convey messages of higher logical type than the contents of those messages. When one person speaks to another the message is usually conveyed in words, but there are additional communications such as gesture, tone of voice and the context of the event. When receiving a message, one has to decide on the categories to which the message belongs. For example, is the message friendly or hostile? At the same time, is it serious or is it a game? Bateson invented the concept of the double bind to describe the confusion that can occur about which category a message should be assigned to. Bateson's work with the families of schizophrenics has produced evidence that putting another person in a double bind is one way people drive each other mad.

While Bateson's work has been fruitful in family therapy, his neglect of the unconscious has meant that his work has largely been ignored by psychoanalysts. Meanwhile the gap between classical theory and what analysts do in sessions, the gap between what we do and what we say we do, is widening all the time.

Freud did not need to think about the social context of his patients' illnesses because the context could be taken for granted. The changes that have taken place in the world in the past fifty years have made Freud's attitudes to family and social life as outdated as the science of his time. On a clinical level there has been enormous development of understanding of the interaction between analyst and patient, but there has not been a comparable change in theory. In his paper 'Does metapsychology still exist?', Arnold Modell (Modell 1981) reviews the main criticisms of Freud's theory that have been made in recent years. He concludes that we still need a two-part metapsychology, an 'I-it' scientific observation and an 'I-thou' hermeneutic approach, presumably expressed in different terms.

Yankelovich and Barrett also provide an excellent critical analysis of Freud's theories in their book *Ego and Instinct* (Yankelovich and Barrett 1970). They are very good on the shortcomings of Freudian theory and the need to connect psychoanalysis with philosophy and natural science. But when they propose a reconstruction of metapsychology they can only say what it should be. They suggest that the concept of meaning should be adopted as a basic concept with the same logical status as tissue states or instinctual drives. Nevertheless, they can only express their ideas about the new metapsychology in classical Freudian terminology.

It is still the rule for analysts to describe their own work with a bias towards agreement with Freud rather than towards establishing the differences. It has not been possible to re-evaluate Freud's work in such a way as to discard the parts that have outgrown their usefulness. Instead a superstructure of psychoanalytical ideas has been developed, in contrast to scientific disciplines which disprove or replace earlier hypotheses. This state of affairs is the result of a category error which would be spotted immediately in a patient. If one heard from the couch that X's theory is so important that all new ideas after X are to be rejected if they contradict X's theory, one would be aware of the error in thinking. The explanation of the persistence of such category errors is to be found in the work of Matte Blanco, which I will discuss presently.

The concepts of double bind and category error provide an opportunity to translate Freud into modern language. Freud's most important discovery was that symptoms have meaning. The process of interpretation can be thought of as trying to identify with increasing accuracy the mistakes in thinking that underlie neurotic symptoms. A neurotic thought is based upon a category error. I hope to show by clinical illustrations that slips of the tongue, misunderstandings in sessions and acting out can be thought of as moments when the patient slips from one category to another, and can take the analyst with him without the analyst noticing.

Matte Blanco also uses Russell's theory of logical types as the mathematical basis for his theory of bi-logic. Bi-logic corresponds very closely to Freud's concept of the primary and secondary processes of thinking. The account I have given of logical typing applies to the secondary process and Matte Blanco's asymmetrical thinking, so called because secondary process thinking makes use of logical categories for the recognition and discrimination of differences. Knowledge of the external world is ordered into categories of space, time and more complex relationships by differentiation into classes or sets. Symmetrical thinking, on the other hand, is equivalent to primary process thinking, where logical categories do not apply. Matte Blanco bases his concept of symmetrical thinking on a part of Russell's theory that deals with an exception to the rule that a class cannot be represented by one of its members. This exception states that when the sets are infinite, the subset is equal to the whole set.

If we consider the mathematical concept of infinity for a moment, we will arrive at the extraordinary discovery that Matte Blanco has found a mathematical means of expressing what we already know about the unconscious. Mathematical sets are ordinarily finite and are a useful way of classifying data, but in abstract terms a set can be infinite. For example, the set of whole numbers, 1, 2, 3, 4 ..., is infinite. From this set a subset can be formed consisting of even numbers, 2, 4, 6, 8 ..., which is also infinite. Then for each number in the set there is one corresponding number in the subset, so that 1 is equivalent to 2, 2 to 4, and so on. While these sets are finite the relationship between the numbers is the obvious one; when the sets are infinite everything changes so that $1 = 2$, $2 = 4$, and so on. This mathematical fact corresponds to the state of affairs that exists in the unconscious, where a part can be equal to a whole. Matte Blanco considers each of the characteristics of the unconscious that Freud described: the absence of time; displacement; replacement of external by internal reality, and the absence of negation. In each case the unconscious process is shown to be the result of the absence of the categories of logical thinking and the presence of the principle of symmetry.

The concept of symmetry is particularly relevant to affects, and Matte Blanco describes experiences of strong emotion as infinite experiences. It is well known that under stress of strong emotion, logical thinking becomes very difficult. I find it helpful to have a mental picture of sets of ideas arranged in an orderly way, with boundaries between the sets. The concept of infinite experience can then be envisaged as the boundaries collapsing so that the sets stretch to infinity. When the categories of logical thinking are broken by symmetrical experience of strong emotion, there is radiation and maximisation of ideas, because the part becomes equal to the whole.

Asymmetrical and symmetrical thinking co-exist in all mental activity in varying proportions. Intellectual activity is mainly asymmetrical, but needs to be supported by an appropriate amount of symmetrical thinking. Matte Blanco describes a number of infinite experiences, of which being in love is the most obvious example. A lover does not see any limits to his love; it is unbounded, and the fact of being in love colours his whole existence. At the same time he has asymmetrical knowledge of the fact that he is in love.

An example of symmetrical experience in analysis is when a patient experiences the analyst as his father in the transference. He knows perfectly well that the analyst is not his father, but in sessions the analyst represents the class of fathers which can be omnipresent, the most unlikely people being part of his feeling about fathers. Material from many different sources can be brought together by a single transference interpretation about the father, which illuminates all the real situations that the patient has been talking about.

Matte Blanco lists other infinite experiences: omnipotence and impotence, idealisation, discouragement, fear and grief. This is not an exhaustive list. Shame and embarrassment also come to mind. The act of thinking is necessarily an asymmetrical experience, but it is inconceivable that any experience of the self, or indeed any mental activity, does not combine symmetrical and asymmetrical elements. The experience of thinking contains symmetrical elements, but the asymmetrical act of thinking extracts meaning from the unconscious by discovering asymmetrical relations in the symmetrical experience. Matte Blanco calls this a translating or unfolding function of the ego, and he considers it to be more important in analysis than the lifting of repression as a means of enlarging the ego.

The concepts of symmetrical thinking and infinite sets amount to a reassessment and re-evaluation of the place of primary process in mental life. I agree with Matte Blanco's assertion that the importance of the ego has been overestimated in the past, to the detriment of psychoanalytical theory.

Another development of the theory of bi-logic is Matte Blanco's exploration of the concept of multidimensional space, which is one aspect of symmetrical thinking. Ideas can be omnipresent, in the same way as threads in a skein, without being all-pervading. This concept explains in part the limitless possibilities of the imagination. For example, speaking of object relations, Matte Blanco writes that at a deep level man does not have relationships with his fellow beings, he *is* his fellow beings (1975: 300).

Reading *The Unconscious as Infinite Sets* produces an indescribable feeling of discovering the truth that one has always known but been unable to express. Under the heading 'Body and Soul' Matte Blanco writes:

> It is interesting to reflect how accurately the old saying 'the body is the mortal wrapping of the spirit' corresponds to what can be said in geometric terms, in which a space of n dimensions can 'envelop' a space of $n + 1$ dimensions: a cube is 'enveloped' by its delimiting planes. The saying suggests that the spirit or soul, whatever that may be, is intuitively conceived as having a greater number of dimensions than the body or matter. (Matte Blanco 1975: 447)

These ideas are of potential value in the clinical situation, where it is a regular occurrence for us to witness the breakdown of the categories of logical thinking under the influence of the transference.

Matte Blanco also provides an explanation of the problems mentioned earlier about psychoanalytical theory. As James Home pointed out (Home 1966), analysts have been the victims of category error in their insistence that psychoanalysis is a science. The application of scientific testing to psychoanalysis is unsatisfactory because we deal with the whole person, including the unconscious. The principle of bi-logic makes it possible to think about this problem in a constructive way and to identify areas in which symmetrical thinking is not being recognised. If a proper value can be assigned to symmetrical experiences they need not be thought of as destructive of logical thinking.

These concepts can be applied to the subject of loyalty to

Freud. There are good historical reasons for Freud's belief that he was a scientist who must formulate his discoveries in terms of the science of his day. Yet from the very beginning analysts have been preoccupied with the poetic and imaginative aspects of his work, and in general we have followed the historical trend in society away from an exclusively scientific attitude. However, at the same time the notion of 'our science' has been clung to tenaciously, in a manner which is unmistakably symmetrical thinking. A simple explanation can be offered. It is not possible to give up a psychological position, or a stage of development, until a possible alternative has appeared. The problem has always been, if psychoanalysis is not a science, what is it?

Now we have the possibility of providing an answer, which is to reformulate Freud's work in modern terms. By the use of Matte Blanco's bi-logic, unconscious symmetrical experience can be understood and expressed in words and mathematical formulae. This translating function involves accepting bi-logic as the central fact of mental life. Previous attempts to find a workable scientific formulation have failed because they did not account for the interrelatedness of primary and secondary processes. Matte Blanco is opening up new fields of enquiry in which emotions may be measured, and statements of great precision may be made about the unity of mental life. One needs to be a mathematician to follow him in all his thinking but the conclusions are not difficult. The essence of his work is the enlargement of horizons in all directions that follows the bringing into relation of the two logics instead of regarding them as incompatible or conflicting.

Matte Blanco's work seems to me to express with beautiful clarity the facts of psychic reality which we all know but have only been able to express clinically. His ideas sweep away all the differences of theoretical outlook and explain how it is that we understand each other across group divisions when patients are being discussed. I think that Bateson and Matte Blanco are describing the same phenomena in different terms. They are both describing a basic pattern of mistakes in thinking. What Matte Blanco calls the use of symmetrical thinking where asymmetrical thinking would be more appropriate, Bateson calls a double bind.

I shall now restate what I have been saying in clinical terms.

The patient is acting upon the assumption that a certain statement is true, while the fact is that a similar, but crucially different, statement is true while the patient's version is false. The difference between the two statements is not appreciated because of the high emotional charge which causes symmetrical thinking to prevail. Under these conditions all sets are infinite, and the capacity for logical discrimination is lost. The child-hood experiences that give rise to mental illness can be described in these terms.

For example, the child of an anxious mother can be in a double bind about turning his attention from his mother to the outside world. At the same time as she encourages him to play, the mother gives the child an unspoken message that it is dangerous to leave her. Instead of the world being an exciting place full of possibilities, new experiences come to have the meaning 'Mummy doesn't like it' so that potentially valuable aspects of the self are labelled bad. Many levels of such experience can be superimposed, with progressive inhibition of some learning capacity, which result in the construction of a set of defences in the adult.

Only when analysis of resistances has uncovered the area of emotional conflict and revealed the double bind, can the differences between the two ideas be identified. An opportunity can then be provided for the patient to learn the difference, which will be learned for the first time. The process of interpretation consists of pointing out the errors in the patient's thinking. When the patient understands his lifelong mistake he will acquire the capacity for more abstract thinking, involving the use of symbols. The capacity for symbolic thinking has been impaired by the process of symptom formation which reduces ideas to a lower category. In other words, the undoing of a double bind presents the patient with alternatives instead of a simple either/or situation. Psychic development consists of the use of progressively higher categories of discrimination, and the acceptance of symbolic substitutes of increasing degrees of abstraction.

To sum up, Bateson and Matte Blanco, from their different viewpoints, are both dealing with the same problem. Bateson's work has proved fruitful in family therapy but it has been largely ignored by analysts because of its disregard of the unconscious as such. Matte Blanco uses conventional terminology to show how Freud's scientific preoccupation with the ego led to his relative neglect of the implications of his discovery of the unconscious. I think Matte Blanco has also provided an explanation of Freud's inability to define the role of the imagination in the individual's adaptation to the external world.

– – –

A clinical illustration is taken from a four-year analysis of a middle-aged professional woman. She has three grown-up children, and a part-time clinical job about which she is extremely conscientious. She came into analysis because of family problems. She had an extremely ambivalent relationship to her mother until her mother's death ten years ago.

When Mrs B was sent away to boarding school at the age of nine, she developed the delusion that her mother was poisonous and she would not touch anything her mother had touched. The symptom implied the unconscious reversal of her denied wish to be close to her mother. Her refusal to wear her new school uniform, which her mother had bought, had the aim of avoiding being sent away. When she started analysis it was obvious that Mrs B was functioning on several levels at once. She had a belligerent manner which challenged me to reject her. She was greatly lacking in self-esteem, and her belligerence concealed an enormous need for reassurance. She acted out in bizarre ways, the main theme being an attempt to prove that she could not be held responsible for her behaviour, and needed to be considered as a special case. She had a brother and sister who were aged twelve and ten when she was born, and her fury at not being able to keep up with them has dominated her life. She was admitted to two mental hospitals during her adolescence. Quite early in the analysis I began to interpret that she was trying to drive me (her mother) mad.

She made impossible demands for a perfect analysis, such as refusing to lie on the couch if the cover was creased. Any indication of the existence of another patient would cause her to walk out. One day she was feeling very cold, but refused to use the blanket because, she said, it radiated cold. She was extremely dependent on me, but expressed her attachment only through continual references to my hostile and rejecting behaviour. She misinterpreted things I said in order to create a framework of rules by which she imagined I conducted the analysis, which was in fact a picture of her paranoid transference. The first significant change occurred when I said that she could only make use of me as a good object by insisting that I was a bad one.

Whatever aspect of her life Mrs B talked about, she compulsively tried to prove that I was wrong and she was right, both by distorting what I said and also by directly attributing ideas to me. Even while accepting an interpretation, and unwittingly giving me confirmation that I was right, she would maintain that I was wrong and create a situation of antagonism. Psychoanalytical jargon was one of her weapons, so I never used technical terms. I coined the phrase 'upside-downness' to describe her state of mind. She gradually accepted this idea as she came to see how she had based her relationship to her mother on hate instead of love.

As everything was paradoxical, progress was measured in terms of getting worse. It was a very long time before she could admit to progress, even though changes were discernible between phases of negative therapeutic reaction. The most important resistance to clinical improvement was the fear that if she got better I would terminate the analysis, a symbolic expression of her fear of being sent away from her mother.

As she became more secure in the relationship, angry scenes became more frequent and acting out more blatant. Several times I had to tell her how obnoxious she was. I felt very uncertain about doing this, but each time the effect was dramatic. She calmed down rapidly and had obviously needed to be told she was behaving badly. Later on I realised she had unconsciously arranged these dramas by making her reported behaviour seem even worse than it was. She needed to be told to stop her temper tantrums, and she had escalated her bad behaviour because I put up with so much. A climax was reached when she shouted at me: 'My mother used to say she loved me and hated my behaviour. I know it wasn't true. She really hated *me*!' I interpreted that she was behaving now as if she was nothing else than her behaviour, and I was able to get her to see the mistake she had made in childhood.

It seems necessary to justify the departure from psychoanalytical technique in telling the patient she is obnoxious. Such an event can only occur spontaneously in a well established transference. An escalation of acting out behaviour indicates a continuing failure of verbal interpretations. When the patient is so disturbed that the analyst's words have no meaning, I think the experience of hearing the analyst interpreting as usual creates a double bind, the signs of interest and concern in the analyst contradicting the negative transference. Breaking the conventions and confronting the patient with the reality of unacceptable behaviour breaks the double bind.

I suggest that her inability to distinguish herself from her behaviour is an important category error. Her idea that she *is* her behaviour makes emotional sense as symmetrical thinking, but if she had been less angry, asymmetrical thinking could have led to the discovery that her mother still loved her even when she was naughty.

Mrs B had a series of dreams at the beginning of her analysis about houses with something wrong with them. She would be living in the basement of a house with other people in the upper rooms, or else the dream houses were uninhabitable for various reasons. In one dream the house was full of corpses. Shortly after the crisis I have described, she dreamed she was stuck fast in a rocky tunnel from which she could only escape by turning into a mist. This was very frightening. There followed a phase of quiet depression, with a series of dreams in which derelict or abandoned houses were brought back into use and daylight was let in. Then she had a strikingly different dream. She was trying to make a telephone call from a telephone which had only a few large deep dialling holes. Someone told her to look down inside these holes, and when she did so she saw that inside each large hole were two or three of the usual dialling holes. She looked again and saw all the people she might ring up. Characteristically she commented that this dream was about the difficulty of communicating with other people. I interpreted it to myself as a good example of the way in which patients' dreams conform to the analyst's expectations. Be that as it may, I do think the dream is a symbolic expression of Mrs B's dawning realisation that change is possible.

When the patient insists that she is her behaviour, she is making a category error. This is a basic situation of a child in a temper tantrum, which can be interpreted in many ways. When Mrs B begins to see herself as a person who is having an experience, instead of being lived by the experience, she moves into a higher category of thinking. After this session she began to be able to compare her own experience with other people's. She had always been good at bringing relevant material from her clinical work, and during good phases I had been able to make interpretations about her and the client simultaneously, which she found illuminating. However, when the negative transference was operating she had to prove me wrong, and used such material to illustrate her uniqueness. After the turning point I have just described, she started to identify with other people in sessions in a useful way.

She told me about a small boy who had many hospital admissions for acute asthma. This boy demanded a toy car from his father every day, and the father gave in because he feared the asthma that frustration might produce. Mrs B recognised that she had been behaving like this boy when she was difficult as a child. In other words she became able to see her childhood in ordinary terms. This incident also explains why it was so effective for me to tell her that she was being obnoxious. I had intuitively broken through my own defences which required me to make correct interpretations, and behaved spontaneously as a parent confronted with a difficult child.

On one occasion I had to change the time of a single session. Although there was no disadvantage in the change, Mrs B constructed an elaborate fantasy that I was fed up with her and wanted to get rid of her. When I interpreted this fantasy she reacted as though I were cutting down the number of sessions per week, not just changing one appointment. I was aware of her scanning my words and only registering those words that fitted in with what she expected to hear. We analysed this event in detail, and I pointed out how she was unable to react normally to the clearing up of a misunderstanding. Instead of thinking 'thank goodness, that's all right' and feeling relieved, she felt as though an abyss had opened. She was able to say that if she fell into the abyss she would stop being special. The further exploration of this experience led to the idea that by reducing all the messages from her mother to a single message of hate, she had become unable to learn.

Another example of this censoring process occurred one day when she was feeling cold, and I asked if she would like me to put the fire on. Without a word she got off the couch and switched on the fire. When I remarked on her difficulty in letting me do anything for her she said in genuine surprise that I had told her to do it herself. In terms of Matte Blanco's bi-logic, the intensity of her ambivalence and fear of rejection make it impossible for her to experience my words realistically. Logical thinking is replaced by symmetrical thinking in which only one idea exists. She edits out of my sentences any words that interfere with the simple message that I am rejecting her.

For example, if I should say: 'You feel angry with me as if I were your mother sending you away to school', as an interpretation of her misunderstanding about the changed session, she would become intensely angry. The interpretation invites the use of asymmetrical thinking to differentiate between present and past, leading to the realisation that I am not rejecting her. Mrs B has to refuse such opportunities, because she has a delusional need to prove that the transference is the only reality and her anger is justified by my rejection of her.

One version of this technique is an unconscious manoeuvre of trying to prove that I said the opposite of what I really said. For example, she took on some extra work to help pay for her analysis. Being poor and being a martyr are important devices for her. She told me that although she was not being paid and was owed £500, she was continuing with this interviewing work. The non-payment was due to an administrative battle between the two authorities involved about who should be paying her. When I made an interpretation about the meaning of her working without payment, she rejected my statement as untrue. She said the money had been provided, and it was only a question of who should do the paperwork. When I pinned her down I was able to show her that she had made a statement contradicting the true facts. In order to get across her message of 'poor little me with such an unsympathetic analyst', she had left out the fact that she knew she would be paid eventually.

There are many occasions when, by leaving out a small word, or by changing the construction of a sentence half-way through, the opposite message is given and the patient remains unaware of the deception. It requires a change of technique, from following the main stream of the session to focusing on a small and apparently irrelevant detail, for such a category error to be analysed.

Some months later Mrs B dreamed about a group of people in a room where a party was in progress. She was showing a male guest around the room. In each corner of the room there was a lavatory and in the middle was a table spread with food. On the table was a lavatory pedestal without a basin, and she was standing on the pedestal defecating and then trying to clear up the faeces and separate it from the food. This dream was used to show her how she is beginning to differentiate between ideas instead of mixing up things that need to be kept distinct. She came to recognise that I had been concerned about her all the time that she had been insisting that I was rejecting her. She spoke about her own inevitable death, and mine, for the first time in the analysis.

At the next session Mrs B was depressed, and talked about the situation at home. She clears up compulsively after the rest of the family. Her husband does the cooking and leaves the kitchen in a mess for her to clear up after the meal. He also listens to music through headphones so he cannot hear what she says. When I linked this material to the dream, she returned to her most vivid childhood memory. She used to sit on her pot in the bathroom playing with bars of variously coloured soap which were kept in a cupboard. She had often recalled this scene as one of being left alone and feeling isolated. On this particular day she told me she used to call out 'I'm red' – short for 'ready' – to tell her mother to come and wipe her. This was the first mention of calling her mother; that is, although her mother was absent she was within call. I asked about her use of 'red' for 'ready' and she told me this referred to traffic lights, because you had to wait for the lights to change to red before you could cross the road. This seems to me a good example of how her pathological thinking developed. The idea that the traffic has to stop before she can go has symbolic meaning for a child who feels the whole world is against her.

Very recently I told Mrs B that I was moving my practice to a much larger house. She said: 'I won't be able to go there', like a frightened child. She talked about stopping analysis when I moved. At the next session she said she had been very childish to get in such a panic, and of course she would come to see me after the move. She said she had had a good dream. She dreamed of a party in my house, and my parents were there and they were kind to her. There was a filing cabinet with the medical records of ten patients in it. She was able to make her own interpretation of not minding that I had other patients now that she feels she belongs in my practice.

— — —

I am suggesting that the ideas of Bateson and Matte Blanco, taken together, provide a new way of formulating psychoanalytical theory based on concepts of logical typing and infinite experiences. I have tried to show how Matte Blanco's ideas throw light on the problem we have all been struggling with, the gap between theory and clinical practice. Rayner (1981) gives an example in his paper of symmetrical thinking experienced during a session. When there is a good interpretation that makes the patient feel his analyst is good, the patient is likely to feel that he is good for his analyst. Rayner makes the important link with Winnicott's work on the baby's fantasy of feeding the mother. This idea is compatible with all theoretical approaches to the mother–infant relationship.

I would like to take symmetrical experience in sessions a stage further, and suggest that infinite experience is the stuff of good analysis. When things are going well the analyst feels at one with the patient. This is most easily described in terms of positive transference and countertransference, but many infinite experiences can be thought of in this way. For example, we all share our patients' grief. Of the less easily shared infinite experiences that Matte Blanco has listed, I find discouragement the most illuminating. The clinical fact that one real-life set-back does produce a radiating and overwhelming feeling of discouragement is a new and useful idea. The concept of infinite experience is also relevant to considerations of shared non-verbal communication in sessions.

In a recent paper entitled 'Strachey's Influence', Darius Ornston (Ornston 1982) describes the subtle difference between

Freud's written German and the English used in the *Standard Edition* of his work. I shall quote Ornston's conclusions:

> By condensing some of Freud's descriptions of his own ideas, Strachey composed a premature technical language which isolated Freud's work from the science of his time, as well as ours, and may have hindered the development of psychoanalytical theory. (Ornston 1982: 424)

In the terms I have been using, this statement can be reformulated to suggest that what Strachey did was to edit out of the original German the symmetrical elements that give Freud's writing its strength and ambiguity. Ornston's work on the difference between Freud in the original and in translation derives from the discussion of this idea by Charles Rycroft in his *Critical Dictionary of Psychoanalysis* (1968a).

Rayner has pointed out the similarity between bi-logic and Suzanne Langer's concept of discursive and non-discursive symbolism, which is fundamental to the work of Milner (1952) and Rycroft (1962). Freud's statement 'where id was, there shall ego be' has little value, on the face of it, for analysts who believe in the importance of the imagination as one of the highest prerogatives of man. Matte Blanco describes his concept of the translating function of the ego as follows:

> When repression is lifted or the unfolding process occurs, there is enlargement of self-awareness. The unconscious is not diminished by this process any more than the size of an object is diminished by being reflected in a mirror or in a million mirrors. The translating function of psycho-analysis draws an inexhaustible supply of asymmetrical relationships from the unconscious to enrich the ego. Because the unconscious is infinite, it is not diminished by this process. (Matte Blanco 1975)

In his last book *Mind and Nature: A Necessary Unity*, Bateson says that if there is a basic unity in the universe, then it is an aesthetic unity (Bateson 1979). As is so often the case, Bateson and Matte Blanco seem to be on the same track. Matte Blanco writes that the basic unity of thinking and emotion seems to be fundamental for the conception of man. The infinite is the meeting point of science and art. He insists that his work is a logical extension of Freud's work and uses the same tools. He believes that Freud did not intend psychoanalysis to be a pure science isolated from other sciences.

To conclude, I have suggested ways in which Matte Blanco's theory of bi-logic can throw light on problems of psychoanalytical theory, particularly the link between theory and clinical practice. While Matte Blanco provides a new way of thinking about such matters, the link with Bateson's work seems to be necessary to achieve a coherent explanation. Both authors are concerned with the basic patterns of the mind. The clarification of theory that is offered by these new ideas could lead to a better integration of psychoanalysis with recent developments in other subjects.

2   Psychoanalysis and Survival*

This chapter continues the themes in Chapter 1 with a discussion of *Wholeness and the Implicate Order* by David Bohm, a theoretical physicist and philosopher. He proposed a systems theory explanation of the nature of the universe which follows from Bateson's notion that mind and evolution are essentially unitary. Bateson's work was part of a new development in human sciences based on systems theory. There have been significant developments in physics, astronomy and evolutionary sciences in recent years as the result of the change to thinking in terms of processes rather than ostensible facts.

Developments in modern physics have rendered the Western tradition of science obsolete. We are accustomed to think of the observer as separate from the objects of consciousness, and the pervasiveness of scientific thinking has led to a very fragmented view of the world. Bohm proposes a new model based on the idea of wholeness. From the idea that what is, is movement, he uses the term 'holomovement' to describe the totality of the universe. His idea of the implicate order is that the universe is enfolded in each of its parts, and any part can unfold to reveal other aspects of reality. Instead of objects and ideas being thought of as separate, as in traditional models of reality, any object or experience can imply all the other aspects of reality.

In contrast to the implicate order there is the explicate order of common-sense reality. The evidence of our senses and scientific observations are relatively stable parts of the holomovement, which can be separated out and have their own validity. Bohm argues that if we live in a self-centred world based on explicate order reality, we will perceive and experience

* First published in the *International Journal of Psychoanalysis*, 1985, 66: 471–80.

the world as fragmented. This view is false because it is based on mistaking our own experience for the true reality. The fragments must be linked in a meaningful way if their significance is to be understood. Each experience or subject of thought contains enfolded within itself the totality of the universe, including both matter and consciousness.

The concept of wholeness is central to Eastern religions and also to Christian mysticism. Bateson and Matte Blanco have both written about wholeness, and their ideas seem to me to be in accord with Bohm's theory of implicate order. The literature on these new models of the mind makes only passing reference to psychoanalysis. The theme of this paper is that it is essential for the survival of psychoanalysis that it should be linked to the evolution of new ideas in other fields.

It occurred to me that Freud could be compared to an explorer, sailing into unknown seas and bringing back a first map of an unknown country. The achievement is enormous and the map is very interesting. Freud's work is the common ground through which we are able to communicate with each other about the unconscious. With the passage of time other discoveries are made, which make it possible to see the original map from previously unsuspected points of view. Because it is such a unique experience to be a psychoanalyst it is difficult for analysts to think about starting to make a new map from scratch, and that is a serious limitation of our thinking.

We are all aware of the growing interest in Eastern philosophy among people who have become disillusioned with Western thinking. In traditional Chinese philosophy the essence of reality or Tao was conceived of as a continual flow between the polar opposites of yin and yang, which are always in dynamic interaction with each other. Yin and yang have many overlapping meanings; yin is feminine, intuitive, responsive and synthesising, while yang is masculine, aggressive, competitive, rational and analytic. In Taoist terms our society is to be considered dangerously unbalanced because of the extreme emphasis on yang qualities. The proliferation of non-scientific interests in recent years is a healthy reaction against a society which feels ever more impersonal. In particular, the ecological movement is an attempt to restore the wholeness of the environment.

Theoretical physics has been the most important source of change in the concept of reality in the twentieth century. Einstein's theory of relativity heralded the end of the era of Newtonian physics. More recently, the discovery of new sub-atomic particles led to the hope that the ultimate units of matter would soon be discovered. This idea is an extreme of yang thinking which inevitably proved to be illusory. As more and more particles were discovered, the traditional scientific distinction between observer and observed had to be abandoned. It seems that particles only exist if they are being observed, and they cannot be said to exist apart from the experimental conditions under which they have been observed. Heisenberg's uncertainty principle represents the fact that the more that is known about the momentum of a particle the less it is possible to know about its position, and vice versa. Physicists came to realise that objective certainty is impossible, and a new model of reality is required. These realisations seem to have found spontaneous expression in terms borrowed from Eastern philosophy. There are now several books explaining subatomic physics to the layman by means of its similarity to Zen.

To summarise what I have been saying, there are important new developments in scientific thinking due to the change to a systems theory approach instead of the traditional view of mechanical sciences. Bateson's concept of mind and nature as essentially unitary has led to new theories of evolution in which macro- and micro-evolution are parts of one self-regulating system. Holistic thinking about the mind requires abandoning the traditional division between scientific and humanistic thinking.

Chapter 1 was an attempt to transcend the limitations of traditional scientific thinking about psychoanalysis by suggest-ing a different relationship between primary and secondary processes. Here I am using Bohm's concept of implicate order to take this process a stage further. In particular, holistic thinking makes it possible to re-examine Freud's attitude to religion. I shall discuss Bohm's ideas in more detail. I shall then discuss Freud's 'The Future of an Illusion' in connection with some recent writing on theology. Then I shall try to show how Bohm's theory applies to psychoanalysis, using my interpreta-tion of Bateson and Matte Blanco.

I shall now describe Bohm's theory of implicate order in more detail. It always takes a long time for the implications of new theories to be understood. For a while the old order can be adjusted to accommodate new information, but this cannot be continued indefinitely. The stress of trying to contain the enormous increase in scientific information in recent years has resulted in the proliferation of new disciplines to deal with interface information. This fragmentation process is in direct opposition to the search for wholeness which Bohm is advocating.

Nuclear physicists had the expectation of discovering the ultimate particles which could be thought of as the building blocks of the universe. What they have discovered makes it impossible to go on thinking in that particular way. If elementary particles can be created, annihilated and transformed into each other under experimental conditions, they cannot be the ultimate particles of matter. The only sensible way to think about them is as part of a flow. The observer and the event observed are part of a larger situation, in which objective information about the thing observed is not possible. It is only possible to describe what was observed under certain conditions. Knowledge too is a process, an abstraction from the total flux which is the ground both of reality and of the knowledge of reality. Bohm uses the word 'holomovement' to describe the totality of our idea of what is. By definition we can only have fragmentary knowledge of the holomovement.

Bohm uses the metaphor of a patterned carpet in which flowers and trees are represented. The relevant way to look at the carpet is to be aware of the pattern, and it is not useful to say that the various motifs are separate objects in interaction. Thinking about patterns instead of units is a basic concept of systems theory, where the concept of a functional organisation is two-faced. It does not matter whether the system under consideration is a person, a social organisation or a machine – it can be thought about in two opposite ways. From one point of view the system is an assemblage of subsystems; from the other it is a unit in a larger system.

Much of Bohm's book is concerned with theoretical physics and the implications of relativity and quantum theory. Relativity makes it impossible to sustain the world view established by Descartes and Newton, which assumes that the world can be divided into separate interacting parts. Quantum theory is equally disruptive of traditional thinking, and a further difficulty exists because it is not possible to reconcile relativity and quantum theory within one frame of reference. The two theories employ incompatible basic concepts. Relativity demands continuity, strict causality and locality; quantum theory requires non-continuity, non-causality and non-locality. Relativity is intimately connected with a mechanistic view of the universe, with which most scientists are still preoccupied. It is still usual for scientists to have an unshakeable faith that the discovery of smaller and smaller particles will reveal the secret of the universe. Meanwhile, ordinary people are increasingly disenchanted with what science has to offer to mankind.

Bohm proposes to give up the idea of a mechanistic order which assumes the separate independent existence of objects, molecules and ideas. Such a view also assumes that the interaction between objects can be seen and measured and that such measurements are the basis of reality. Bohm calls this world view the explicate order. His world view is an implicate order, in which reality is enfolded in complex ways and can be unfolded and made manifest. The explicate order of common-sense reality is a relatively stable part of the total reality or holomovement.

The mechanistic view of reality which we all share is extremely difficult to give up, particularly since it has been reinforced by the invention of photography. Now that we can see photographs of things that cannot be seen with the naked eye, the structure of matter seen under high-power magnification can mistakenly be thought to be the appropriate way to conceive it. Obviously, scientific thinking is not to be abandoned; what needs to change is the idea that a scientific view is the proper or only way to view reality.

The implicate order based on the concept of wholeness reconciles the incompatible elements in relativity and quantum theory. Bohm illustrates implicate order by using the example of the hologram. If coherent light from a laser beam is passed through a half-silvered mirror on to a photographic plate, a three-dimensional image of an object in its path can be obtained. The mirror reflects half the light on to the object while the other half reaches the plate directly, so that an interference pattern is formed on the plate. The two images combined on the plate may produce a pattern which is meaningless to the naked eye, but when the plate is illuminated by laser light, a three-dimensional image is produced, which can be seen from many points of view. The pattern on the plate has an implicit relation to the illuminated image. If one part of the plate is illuminated an image of the entire object is still produced, but from a restricted point of view, with poorer definition. The implicate order consists of a similar enfolding of parts within the whole, so that each part of reality implies all the other parts without discontinuity.

Another way of conveying the idea of implication is to think of putting one's eye to a telescope; the whole landscape is enfolded at that point. Accepting the idea of a new order of reality requires an imaginative leap away from the old order of cause and effect. The separate existence of ordinary observable phenomena, which Bohm calls the explicate order, is a special case of a more general set of implicate orders.

The way we can imagine the world to be from the evidence of our senses is an explicate order, distinguished by the selection of relatively stable and recurrent elements which are outside each other. This has been the basis of a mechanistic approach to reality and of the assumption that such elements *are* the basic reality. The implicate order, on the contrary, starts with the undivided wholeness of the universe, and the task of science is then to discover the parts as approximately separable and recurrent, and therefore describable in terms of explicate order as relatively autonomous entities.

Quantum theory indicates that matter cannot be broken down into series of separate related particles and fields. Quantum theory supposes particles to be fragments of a multidimensional reality which is not totally comprehensible in terms of interactions between the particles. To demonstrate this higher order of reality we can think about a tank of fish in a television studio. Imagine an oblong tank with two cameras, A and B, photographing adjacent sides of the tank at right angles to each other. Imagine two screens side by side projecting images from the two cameras. A fish in side view on screen A will appear head on at the same moment on screen B. The viewer will be

aware that the images are of the same fish because the
movements are in some way the same on the two screens.
Neither screen gives the total reality of the fish; each is a
projection in two dimensions of a three-dimensional reality
which is beyond both. There is already a widespread intuitive
awareness that television has brought us a new order of reality.
There are numerous feature films where important scenes
about incompatible views of reality are set in a television studio
against the background of the banks of monitor screens.

Bohm quotes experiments in which two atoms are made to
combine to form a molecule. Under most conditions each atom
can be seen to exist in three-dimensional space, but it is
possible to think of them as projections of a six-dimensional
reality. If the molecule is made to disintegrate so that the atoms
are separate and distant and do not interact, they can be found
to relate to each other in a similar way to the images of the fish
on the television screens. The two three-dimensional projections corresponding to the two atoms may have a relative
interdependence of behaviour. Under such conditions they can
be described in ordinary three-dimensional terms of the explicate order, as relatively independent interacting particles. More
generally they will show typical non-correlation of behaviour,
which implies that they do not exist in the same three
dimensions. A six-dimensional description is required to
account for the behaviour of such particles.

The implicate order is to be thought of as a process of
enfoldment and unfolding in multidimensional space. The
dimensionality of the universe is effectively infinite. The
explicate order consists of relatively stable independent sub-
totalities unfolded from the total holomovement.

The difference between the mechanistic and implicate orders
is like the difference between a living organism and a machine.
The parts of a machine are made separately and can be taken
apart and reassembled. The parts of a living organism have
grown in the context of the whole organism in its environment,
and they cannot be separated. The laws of nature can be
explained in a more satisfactory way in implicate order terms. A
forest can be thought of as a stable entity, because although
trees are dying and regrowing, in the long term the tree
population remains stable. The death and replacement of one

tree is only of local significance. The seed from which the tree grows has very little to contribute to the final form of the tree, which depends on soil, water and sunlight. The seed provides the DNA which informs the matter of the environment so that inanimate material is transformed into a living tree. We are used to thinking of living matter and inanimate matter as completely separate, but this is only true in explicate order thinking. The environment will continue as inanimate without a seed, but there is no division between inorganic molecules which are incorporated into a plant and those which are not. A molecule of carbon dioxide which crosses a cell boundary to enter a leaf does not 'come alive' at that moment, nor does the molecule of oxygen released at the same moment 'die'. It only makes sense to think of the plant and the environment as a totality. As I have already described, the technique of isolating the phenomena we wish to study is explicate order thinking.

Unfortunately, psychoanalysts are still suffering from confusion due to the continuation of mechanistic thinking, although dynamic processes have long been recognised as a more appropriate model. Marjorie Brierley wrote about psychoanalysis as process theory in 1944. Although her work is not often quoted nowadays, her influence is implicit in the thinking of the Independent Group of the British Psychoanalytical Society (Brierley 1932, 1944). This is discussed in more detail in Chapter 3. This paper is part of that tradition.

The most difficult problem in establishing a new order of thought is the relationship of consciousness to objective reality. Descartes explained the relationship between them by making God responsible for both, since He had created both mind and matter. Since the part played by God has been removed from the scheme of things, the Cartesian tradition has collapsed.

The implicate order provides a means of uniting matter and consciousness which is very similar to modern theological conceptions of God. Bohm goes into great detail to explain consciousness in implicate order terms. Recent work on brain function suggests that the way information is stored in brain cells can be described more successfully by the hologram analogy than by traditional scientific means. Bohm uses the experience of listening to music to demonstrate that consciousness is a flow of momentary events, each of which implies what has gone before and what is yet to come. Explicit order descriptions of separate moments fail to explain the actual experience, which is that what is, is movement. Much of the difficulty is because time is conceived as linear in explicate order thinking, consciousness being a series of moments succeeding each other. If one thinks in implicate order terms about the flow of thought, subjective experience consists of a series of inter-mingling and interpenetrating elements in different degrees of enfoldment, all present together. The sharp break between immediate experience and abstract logical thought is thereby overcome. The possibility is presented of a flowing movement from immediate experience to logical thought and back again, and an end to the fragmentation of thinking.

The next point to consider is memory. The process of thinking is not just a representation of the external world. The way we experience the world is greatly influenced by memory; we see what we expect to see. Thinking makes an important contribution to the manifest world by providing the strong element of stability and predictability which we take for granted. Against this stable background, the changing flow of experience is seen as fleeting impressions which are arranged on the stable background which we call reality. Piaget's work on the begin-nings of consciousness showed that rational thinking about space, time and causality have to be learned by the infant, whereas the awareness of movement is present from birth (Piaget 1956).

Bohm proceeds further to show that matter and conscious-ness have a common ground in the holomovement. Memory is a special case of the flow of momentary events, in that past moments are recorded in the brain cells, which are indubitably a part of matter. Memories can be said to be enfolded in the brain in the same way as traces of past events are recorded in rocks as strata and fossils. Cameras, tape-recorders and computers record events which can be unfolded from film or tape in a way not essentially different from the way the history of the earth can be reconstructed from the fossil record. This means that the explicate order of reality is not essentially different from matter and they are different aspects of the same totality. Ordinary consciousness and ordinary appreciation of the world are both part of the holomovement. The relationship between them can be considered in terms of the relationship between mind and body. Instead of familiar concepts of psychosomatic interaction with mind and body thought of as separate, a statement in implicate order terms would be that the mind enfolds the whole of matter and the body in particular. Similarly the body enfolds not only the mind but in some sense the entire material universe.

If one can think in terms of multidimensional reality, then the awareness that we have can be thought of as projected into lower dimensional elements. The ultimate reality enfolds all experience into a higher dimensionality which is infinite. I want to suggest that Bohm's theory is a more easily understood statement of the same idea as Bateson's view that mind and evolution are essentially unitary. In 1970, Bateson pointed out the urgency of the need for a shift from traditional thinking to cybernetic thinking. He saw that the unit of survival in evolution is the flexible organism plus its environment. This recognition led him to important truths about the necessity for healing the splits that exist in many areas of human life. Since then the science of cybernetics has proliferated without regard to the human environment, and the divisions in the world confirm Bateson's view of the inevitable self-destructiveness of systems that proliferate in a self-limited way. These ideas are entirely in accord with Bohm's view of the limitations of explicate order thinking.

Psychoanalysis is the science of the unconscious and it has lost its dynamism. The evolutionary process will render psychoanalysis obsolete unless we can develop a new mode of expression of our knowledge. The idea of a new order is something that can only be glimpsed at present, and any definitive form must be some way in the future. The new order can be grasped imaginatively by people who can combine primary and secondary process thinking in order to overcome the problems of using conventional terminology to describe the modern world. It seems to me that what is required is a shift into a higher logical type of thinking, as Bateson described. It is often forgotten that a double bind can lead to creativity as well as illness. Bateson transformed our thinking about interpersonal relationships with the concept of the double bind. An even more dramatic change could be brought about by implicate order concepts. Bohm's model of the mind provides a means to combine scientific thinking with the powerful emotional force of the alternative cultures that have developed out of young people's disenchantment with society. If the yin is indeed in the ascendant and likely to supersede the yang, it will be important for a new concept to be available as a focus for developing ideas. If integration rather than fragmentation is to occur, a theory such as implicate order will be required.

I hope I have demonstrated that it is no longer realistic for psychoanalysis to be looking backwards to Freud. It is an urgent matter to reformulate our knowledge of the unconscious in ways which can make sense of the changes in scientific thinking.

In his recent book *Freud and Man's Soul*, Bruno Bettelheim (Bettelheim 1983) asserts that Freud had a secular view of spiritual matters which included all the qualities which are associated with the word 'soul'. He disagrees with the translators of the *Standard Edition*, who felt obliged to use an alternative word to soul out of consideration for Freud's views on religion. Whatever the rights and wrongs of translation, Bettelheim would have us believe that something has been lost when we use the word 'psyche' and take little interest in religious experience.

In 'The Future of an Illusion', Freud (Freud 1927) described religion as the obsessional neurosis of mankind. He ended with the words, 'It would be an illusion to suppose that what science cannot give us we can get elsewhere.' The paper is cast in the form of an imaginary dialogue with an opponent who champions the cause of religion against Freud's rational argument. The religious view is represented by the god of Necessity, providing mankind with an illusion of security. Freud's god is *Logos*, appropriately translated here as Reason. There is no sign that either Freud or the translators considered the fact that the first association many people have to the word *logos* is 'In the beginning was the word.'

At this distance in time it is possible to see what Freud could not see: that his affirmation of his belief in the science of psychoanalysis was a belief of the same order as religious belief, so that there is no discrepancy in the two uses of *logos*. Freud expressed the hope that Reason would lead to a better world in the distant future. He added, 'If experience should show ... that we have been mistaken, we will give up our expectations.' He also wrote in this paper, 'Nothing can withstand reason and experience, and the contradiction which religion offers to both is all too palpable.' Freud's attacks on organised religion are easy to justify, but he was less successful in dismissing individual religious experience. The ideas expressed by his imaginary opponent could be taken as an expression of Freud's sadness at abandoning religion. One wonders how much he knew about Christian theology, and whether he knew that 'The Word was made flesh and dwelt among us.' It seems likely that his attitude to religion was based on the Jewish tradition in which he grew up, which it is surely reasonable to compare to an obsessional neurosis.

Now I shall return to the idea mentioned in Chapter 1, that Freud did not sufficiently value the role of the primary process in mental life, in the hope of arriving at a world view which gives a central role to the unconscious and imagination. By doing so I hope to resolve some of the difficulties with which Freud was faced in this area.

Bohm is a philosopher as well as a physicist, and he refers to Freud in his book. He compares his own view of the unconscious to the oceanic feeling. Matte Blanco is emphatic that his own work on the unconscious is a direct continuation of Freud's work, and I find his claim convincing. Matte Blanco's concept of multidimensional space is virtually the same as Bohm's concept of the infinite dimensionality of the holomovement. It is interesting that Bohm has derived his ideas from theoretical physics, but not as surprising as it seems at first sight. All scientific theories are products of the human mind, and are part of an ongoing process of attempts to explain the universe. The idea of the holomovement as the ultimate reality and the explicate order as everyday reality is not essentially different from a religious concept of revealed truth which has to be sought beyond the world of appearances. The general significance of these ideas is that imagination, or primary process, is the basis of reality. To put it another way, 'We are such stuff as dreams are made on.'

If one can detach oneself from the conventional framework of space and time, it is possible to take a different view of familiar experiences, which is immediately more satisfying. We are all familiar with the liberating effect on a patient when a session has offered an alternative to the rigid way the patient has been thinking. The same thing can happen in everyday life. The common-sense law of local causes is the first casualty of quantum theory. We all have experiences which are not explicable by the law of local causes, but we usually explain them away and keep our common sense. Consider the concept of linear time. It is possible to conduct a session or a conversation in which events follow each other in a straight line, so that each person is replying to what the other has just said. This is a very inadequate description of a session, and one of the reasons why it is so difficult to report sessions convincingly is that the events are not linear. Both minds are ranging to and fro over time, and it is not uncommon for the analyst's association to a patient's words to anticipate what the patient is on the point of saying.

Similarly, when looking at a picture, or watching a play, the mind is free of the restrictions of time. It may be objected that I am merely describing imagination. Here is an example of experiences over the last fifty years. When I was a child, toy trains were mechanical and had to be wound up. Then electric trains arrived and seemed to run by magic. Then came remote control, and another seemingly magical escape from the mechanical world. Nowadays young children are becoming familiar with computers before they can read, and use them to acquire basic skills. All these developments have become part of our thinking over a period of time which can be seen as linear, but the nature of the world has not changed. We can look back and remember a world without electronics. We can look forward in imagination and know that similar changes will occur in the future. Yet on a far more important level of experience we know that we are part of a universe in which human discoveries are of little account.

Surely it must be the case that the human mind is part of the biological unity of nature and any attempt to stand outside the current of thought is doomed to failure. Attempts at preserving old ways of thinking will not do. Psychoanalysis represents a significant area of knowledge which needs to be translated from the now dead world of mechanical science into the developing world of supra-rational thought. In this context the fact that Freud was a Viennese Jew is of historical interest, but of little value compared with the importance of his discoveries.

I think it is possible to connect the scientific thinking I have been discussing with trends in modern theology. God has been transformed from the traditional 'God out there' into the basic stuff of the universe, the ground of our being. God is the basic energy that transforms thought into creativity. The idea of God as continuous flux was part of early Christianity, and similar ideas are common in Eastern religions. God as unknowable and ineffable is a comparable statement to Bohm's notion of the holomovement as essentially unknowable and unmeasurable.

In *The Duality of Human Existence*, David Bakan wrote:

> scientific and religious enquiry are not so separate as modern thinking commonly assumes. In recent centuries science may have seemed to replace the Judaeo-Christian tradition so that people felt they had to make a choice between one or the other. Both science and religion assume that the ultimate reality is different from the manifest. The mistake that both approaches can make is to regard their discoveries as fundamental when they can only be part of the unknown made manifest. Science has commonly been guilty of this in our time. (Bakan 1966)

Psychoanalysis is guilty of the same error when it fails to connect with other branches of knowledge.

In Chapter 1 I drew attention to the fact that both Bateson and Matte Blanco have written about unity and infinity. Matte Blanco wrote that infinity is a way of thinking about God; Bateson foresaw a need to find a definition of the sacred. He wrote that if there is a unity in the universe, it must be an aesthetic unity. The theologian Don Cupitt expresses similar ideas in his book *Taking Leave of God* (Cupitt 1980). He argues that modern science, and the possibility of autonomy for the mass of individuals in free countries, have made it impossible to believe in 'a God out there'. Like other contemporary theologians, he regards religious dogma as a myth. His description of the struggle of the individual towards autonomy is familiar to us from what we hope for as the end result of analysis. His title is taken from Meister Eckhart: 'Man's last and highest parting occurs when for God's sake, he takes leave of God.' Surely this is a comparable statement to the idea of accepting one's own reality through psychoanalysis.

Cupitt surveys the history of Jewish and Christian theology. He describes a historical process of gradual internalisation of religious institutions. There is a progressive development to-wards a more inward spiritual concept instead of an outward form. The explicit notion of order represented by the rules of the Church is replaced by personal beliefs about the ordering of one's own life. The process of demythologising and internalising is described in the Bible. Jehovah is originally thought of as fighting on Israel's side and giving victory in battle. In the New Testament the struggle against evil has been internalised as the spiritual battle within the individual. Literal notions of hell, resurrection and the last judgement have undergone a similar transformation.

The religious concern is not for verbal formulae, but for a state of the self and a way of being. Cupitt regards St Paul's thought about the resurrection as existential. He sees historical concern about the resurrection as ludicrously misplaced; people who engage in such activities are misunderstanding the problem by applying modern language concepts. For example, the word 'fact' has a scientific meaning now which was not available in the first century. Cupitt sees the task of the theologian as extracting meaning from the myth. He quotes Bultmann:

> Every talking about presupposes a standpoint apart from what is being talked about. But there can be no standpoint apart from God, and for that reason God does not permit Himself to be spoken of in general propositions, universal truths which are true without reference to the concrete existential situation of the one who is doing the talking. (Cupitt 1980)

Bultmann regards Freud's notion that God is a projection of the individual's father as 'shallow enlightenment'.

Religion for Cupitt is not metaphysics but salvation, and salvation is a state of the self. In his modern view of Christianity, attempts to retain the New Testament are doomed, except in a symbolic sense. The love of God is a disinterested love. The pursuit of the religious ideal needs no justification. One must seek higher purity and intensity of consciousness because consciousness itself, and perhaps all biological life, is such a teleological striving. God is needed as a myth to live by, but the individual can transcend the myth. Cupitt is making a statement of essential Christian experience which is an avowal of hope and a moral code at the same time; it includes cosmic awe and disinterested love.

Spontaneous religious experience can be considered as a continuation of primary biological knowledge. Faith is an expression of inner certainty. It seems to me that the implicate order has exactly the same meaning – glimpses of the true order give us the idea of the unknowable holomovement which equals God, and which we feel part of when we are in a state of wholeness. It should be possible to express psychoanalytical ideas in this way. Genital love is presumably disinterested love, the capacity to bring up children without selfish damage to the unfolding of the implicate order in the life of each child.

The implicate order is a concept which is helpful in understanding double binds, which can be more complex than the explanation given by Bateson. Even though a double bind can be reduced to a pair of contradictory messages, the power of the bind is due to the implicit meaning enfolded in the relationship of the people concerned. The change produced in a patient can be thought of in the same way. The interpretation of personal experience on a simple level of transference and family relationships has meaning on may other levels, which can unfold once the new idea is understood by the patient.

It does not seem to me to matter very much if objections are made to Bohm's implicate order as a model for a new way of thinking. The important point is that many people have been trying to get beyond the limitations of conventional ideas, but there has been great difficulty in combining new theories. Bateson seems to have been the first to make a breakthrough with his use of logical typing to arrive at the double bind theory of human behaviour. Bateson and Bohm both make use of systems theory, but neither of them has been directly concerned with the study of the unconscious. They have not tackled Freud's major problem, that the unconscious is not amenable to logic.

In his book on creativity, Sylvano Arieti (Arieti 1976) proposes a tertiary mental process to describe the combining of primary and secondary processes in successful creative thinking. This idea could be useful in applying implicate order to psychoanalysis. Primary and secondary process thinking are different in kind, and a new method of combining ideas is needed to describe their interaction. If I am right in my understanding of Bohm, the holomovement is the primary process, and the unique human achievement is the ability to extract useful explicate order reality from the holomovement in the form of secondary process thinking. The danger that this ability carries with it is that human beings can and do become alienated from their grounding in the natural world. The development of creative thinking, a tertiary mental process, is our evolutionary potential and the requirement for solving the problems of living in the world.

To summarise what I have been saying, Bohm's theory of implicate order has profound significance for psychoanalysis. His concept of the holomovement can be recognised as the unconscious, the ultimate reality, from Freud's description and from Matte Blanco's elaboration of it in multidimensional space. Implicate order throws light on the problem Freud faced when formulating his theories, hampered as he was by the limitations of nineteenth-century mechanistic science. Scientific formulations about the mind are valid as long as it is recognised that they are explicit order phenomena, to use Bohm's term, and therefore incomplete.

Analysts know very well that intellectual formulations are inadequate. Freud was pointing out all along that consciousness was not enough. The proliferations of theory that we have been suffering from are the result of trying to accommodate new ideas in an outmoded theoretical form. There is an enormous amount of information available about the human mind, but it is all in fragments. This is because the old order of thought cannot keep up with new ideas which are developing all the time, which need to be connected with each other in new ways. If the different branches of knowledge can be viewed as explicate order phenomena unfolded from the total holomovement of human thought, it becomes possible to use connections which have been rejected in the past as irrational and unscientific. In particular, meaning is just as valid as proof, and thought needs to be anchored in one person's experience.

Freud's work takes on a new dimension when viewed in this way. The subtle unfolding of meaning in the life of the individual, and the acceptance of the imagination as the core of the self, make much better sense than the mechanical model Freud was obliged to use. The escape from linear time which is now possible means that the past unfolds in a new way from each point of view. To think about Freud's work in this way is to marvel again at the magnitude of his achievement in charting the unconscious. It is also to see how the proper understanding of mental life has had to wait for a new context of thinking in order for us to understand Freud's historical limitations.

3   A Concept of Femininity: Sylvia Payne's 1935 Paper Reassessed*

In recent years a great deal has been written about femininity, but Sylvia Payne's paper is hardly ever mentioned. This seems to me to be unfortunate, because her attitude to femininity has been handed down in the Independent Group of the British Psychoanalytical Society. Although unrecognised, her influence is often implicit.

In the 1930s the British Psychoanalytical Society was small enough for everyone to know each other and exchange ideas. The writings of Marjorie Brierley, Ella Sharpe, Sylvia Payne and John Rickman can be thought of as the nucleus of what was later to become the Independent Group within the Society. These writers had a common cultural background at a time when educated people had not begun to think of themselves as specialists. They did not have separate categories for their knowledge of medicine, English literature, psychoanalysis, and so on. In that intellectual environment Marjorie Brierley wrote about psychoanalysis as process theory as a natural extension of Freud's work (Brierley 1932).

Sylvia Payne's paper on femininity deserves to be read as a record of the dynamic thinking at that time which has been overshadowed by later developments in theory. Her starting point was Brierley's notion that a psychological definition of femininity might have to be made in terms of integration. This is a development of Brierley's idea of psychoanalysis as process

* First published in the *International Review of Psychoanalysis*, 1987, 14: 237–44.

theory, which conceives of female functioning in holistic terms. Brierley expressed her agreement with Payne's work in the second of her two papers about women, in which she tried to integrate her own views with Freud's formulations about early female development. Brierley did not include these two papers on female sexuality when she collected and revised her published work as her book *Trends in Psychoanalysis* (Brierley 1951). I hope to show in the course of this chapter why I think Brierley failed to achieve a synthesis of her own views with Freud's. Payne's paper is incompatible with Freud's theory of female sexuality. She puts forward a theory of female development in which Freud can clearly be seen to be describing pathology, not normal development. I shall summarise Payne's paper and discuss it from a holistic point of view. An account of a single session will follow, to illustrate the final discussion.

Payne begins with Brierley's notion that the basis of ego function is the integration and co-ordination of conflicting male and female elements in the personality. In considering the sexuality of women, she points out that the sexual function is only partly fulfilled in the sexual act. The psychic reaction to all aspects of child-rearing is profound, and can overshadow sexual activity. She lists the demands normally made on an adult woman, and the psychic qualities required to fulfil these demands. After listing the demands, she discusses their relationship to feminine functioning. I shall give the list in full, and then summarise her discussion.

The requirements are:

1. Receptivity rather than passivity.

2. The capacity to tolerate and adapt to repeated variations in secondary narcissism.

3. The capacity (not exclusively female) to sublimate trends depending on opposite sex elements in the personality without destroying or inhibiting her real sex.

4. A willingness to receive and retain, co-ordinated with a wish to give out, in a pattern which is inherent in the nature of the female sexual function.

In discussing the first requirement, receptivity, Payne questions Freud's view of the path taken by the libido in a baby girl. She suggests that the constellation of penis envy described by Freud is a pathological outcome. She quotes Joan Riviere, from a review of Freud's 'New Introductory Lectures': 'It is not a credible view of woman, and even Freud has not always looked at woman thus' (Riviere 1934).

Payne stresses the underlying rejection of femininity in women who have a phallic organisation of the self. She accepts Melanie Klein's view that in the earliest stages a girl's deepest fear is of the inside of her body being robbed or destroyed. Payne confirms Klein's connection of oral sucking with vaginal sucking, both from observations made of infants and from the sexual experiences of adult patients. She points out the pathological twist involved in Freud's statement that the wish to incorporate the father's penis is a wish to be male.

In discussing the second requirement, the capacity to undergo repeated variations in secondary narcissism, Payne surveys the whole field of object relations in terms of oral and anal fantasies. At each stage she contrasts fantasies belonging to a good object relationship, which facilitate further healthy development, with the pathological outcome if a good relationship is lacking. There is nothing surprising in her description; the most striking qualities are the emphasis on the social implications of the various psychological positions, and her recognition of how impossible it is to separate normal and abnormal in the adult. She recognises that many so-called pathologies are socially useful if not taken to extremes. She ends this discussion with a summary of the reassurance a mother may gain when she nurses her baby successfully:

1. In so far as the child represents a substitute for the superego, she reconciles herself with it.

2. She has a successful unconscious relationship with a substitute for the introjected parental image.

3. She proves that her infantile active and passive oral fantasies are not destructive in character.

4. The unconscious identification of breast and penis satisfies her penis envy and thus diminishes her sense of inferiority.

5. She successfully fulfils the final stage of her feminine reproductive function by 'giving out'.

6. The psychical libidinal losses experienced in the act of birth are partially compensated for by the identification between child and mother in the act of nursing.

Payne writes that the third requirement, the sublimation of opposite sex elements, involves the primary masculine elements in the woman's personality. This needs to be differentiated from the masculine complex, or reactive identification with the father in a flight from femininity. She sees the analyst's task as comparison of the significance of the various determinants.

The fourth requirement, the most essential feminine capacity, is the co-ordination of a wish to receive coupled with a wish to give out. Payne says this capacity is necessary for the performing of all a woman's biological functions. She discusses orgasm, birth and lactation in relation to this capacity. She lists the factors that can inhibit orgasm as biting fantasies, mistaken identification of the vagina and anus, sadistic birth fantasies in which the clitoris is identified with the sadistic internal object which the baby represents, so that clitoral orgasm is inhibited; and projection of sadistic fantasies on to the sexual partner, leading to frigidity. There is a similar discussion of the pathology of childbirth and lactation.

In her concluding paragraphs Payne states that the flexibility required for mature sexual functioning is also required if the mother is to meet the demands of the growing child. When this flexibility is absent, 'the chief interest is in the child as a possession. Independence of the child cannot be tolerated, owing to the narcissistic injury which would be incurred.'

Payne's last reference is to Ella Sharpe's paper on rhythm and pattern in psychic life (Sharpe 1935). She writes that in considering these phenomena, which parallel the physical rhythms of the body such as breathing and heartbeat, we are on the threshold of an unexplored land better known to oriental philosophers. Here again her thinking is prophetic of the way attitudes have changed in recent years.

Charles Rycroft pointed out that when Freud described the primary process he

> unwittingly became involved in a paradoxical activity when he tried to formulate in words the nature of a type of thinking which is essentially non-verbal and which is, therefore, of necessity falsified by being put into words. But as a rationalist and a scientist he really had no option but to try. (Rycroft 1985: 263)

Rycroft extends Freud's description of the unconscious in negative terms to suggest that the same negative qualities are characteristic of the literary imagination. This view of the imagination was the source of my idea that the unconscious mind is the same thing as David Bohm's holomovement, the ground of all that is (see Chapter 2). I am now going a step further to suggest that the primary process is feminine and the secondary process is masculine. The two modes together represent the bisexuality of the human mind.

Constructing a theory of femininity is a secondary process activity which inevitably describes the feminine in secondary process (or, as I would have it, masculine) terms. The subjective has to be objectified when we describe analysis in words, but this is not true of the experience of the session. Although Freud thought of himself as a scientist, he was writing imaginatively about his patients. The concept of male and female thinking going on in patient and analyst all the time could lead to a new dimension in our understanding of Freud. With a multidimensional approach, similar ideas can be re-combined in an integrative way which provides an escape from the 'either/or' type of thinking. From this point of view Payne and Brierley's awareness of the integrative aspect of feminine thinking is a landmark in the development of holistic thinking about psychoanalysis. Implicate order provides the means to transcend the limitations of scientific and common-sense thinking so that it becomes possible to think of primary and secondary process as complementary female and male aspects of the mind.

Freud wrote that in health the two mental processes are indivisible, and their separate operation can only be discerned in illness. Payne's idea of femininity as an integrative process is in line with this, in contrast to the splitting into constituent parts which is involved in a scientific analysis. In holistic terms the Oedipus complex can be expanded to include multiple identifications with male and female aspects of both parents, and with other significant figures such as grandparents and teachers. This kind of thinking seems to me to be taken for granted by many Independent Group analysts who are not aware of Payne's influence or the existence of her paper.

Payne retained Freud's theory of infantile sexuality but she was not restricted by it. She used Freud's stages of development within a broader scheme of her own in which the growth of the child as a whole person, from infantile egocentricity to adult autonomy, is never lost sight of. Although she does not say so explicitly, Payne is writing symbolically throughout. Infantile dependence is symbolised by the oral stage, problems of power and self-control by the anal stage, and infantile genitality by the phallic phase. The various pathologies of sexual development are partial failures of symbolic transformation. Payne stresses, above all, reality testing which brings awareness of other people, particularly those of the opposite sex, and the role of the sexes in society. In other words, in healthy development the earliest experiences are integrated into a sense of a self who experiences relationships. If there is not enough good experience, or if there is object loss, there is a failure of symbolisation and infantile experience remains concrete.

What I have described so far is familiar and the holistic aspect is unimportant. I want to pursue the holistic line of thought to suggest that with a concept of male and female thinking separate from male and female bodies, mental bisexuality can be separated from physical gender. There is hardly ever any doubt about the sex of a child; it is in our minds that we are bisexual. There is no childhood experience which has a predictable outcome. Basic experiences, such as the birth of a sibling, can have unlimited consequences depending on the state of mind of the child and on environmental factors.

The concept of male and female thinking explains how opposite sex elements are integrated into the personality, as Payne described, without damage to the sexual identity of the adult. The concept also provides the possibility of making a theoretical distinction between the normal and the abnormal. Freud gave a clear account of the transition from sucking the breast to vaginal sucking, with fellatio as an intermediate stage. We do not hear very much about the normal development of this fantasy. There must be many women who have identified with their fathers through a fantasy of incorporating his penis in a healthy way. In normal women the fantasy may be unconscious, but whether it is accessible or not, it does not give rise to anxiety. It cannot be the fantasy as such that gives rise to symptoms. As Payne indicates, it must be the relationship of the fantasy to the whole psychic organisation. Hysterics have symptoms because the fantasy is concretised and unavailable for symbolic transformation into whole person experience. The relative absence of good experience in the hysterical personality means that the primitive sadistic fantasies have not been modified by reality testing.

Another consequence of thinking in terms of psychic bisexuality is the possibility of thinking about a child having masculine and feminine experiences simultaneously. With patients we are usually aware of the failure of integration of the two kinds of experience, and the analytic process leads to a decrease in the extent to which the patient is out of touch with the self.

Women patients often have difficulty in talking about their sexuality because of concretised fantasies, such as feeling that the body is disgusting, because a sense of personal integrity is lacking. In such girls the development of identity was impaired by the mother's inability to see the child as a separate person. Payne describes this in her discussion of the need for flexibility of adaptation. She writes that failure in this capacity leads to treating the child as a possession. Payne knew that little girls have an instinctive knowledge about the inside of their bodies which is the basic female identity, and defences are concerned with protecting the inside from attacks. On this basis, Freud's theory of penis envy is the psychopathology of women who have been damaged in their primary feminine feelings.

The concept of male and female thinking also clarifies the theory of hysteria. The male elements in a woman's mind, and in particular her identity as represented by a phallic symbol, are theoretically the same as a man's. Although the sex of the person cannot be disregarded clinically, and the overall role of the opposite sex elements must be different in men and women, it could be helpful to make this connection. It is in respect of her identity that a hysterical woman feels castrated, and it is the result of a category error that the psychopathology centres on an actual penis. The ancient connection of hysteria with the womb fits in with this theory, since a male hysteric has the same kind of defect of self-esteem, and his feminine thinking can be deformed as a result of the same processes that we are familiar with in women.

The phallic woman can have her whole personality organised around a fantasy penis and competitive behaviour. This narcissistic state interferes with the development of a sense of reality. Payne says that in such women there is always an underlying rejection of femininity, and the relationship between mother and child must be thoroughly analysed before the importance of the masculine complex can be estimated. I would add to this that the phallic behaviour is the basis for competitiveness with other phallic women, particularly the mother, just as much as with men.

To sum up my interpretation of Payne's holistic approach in the bisexual terms I am using, it seems to me that a woman cannot organise her femininity in an adult way without a phallic symbol, and in the same way a man cannot achieve maturity without acceptance of his own femininity.

– – –

I shall now give a clinical illustration from a session with a woman in her late forties whom I shall call Louise. My aim is to demonstrate the dynamic process in the session, so I shall give only the essential information.

Louise was the only member of her working-class family to go to a grammar school. She won a scholarship to art school, but her parents would not let her go because it was not a good financial prospect. She worked as a secretary instead. Louise had attended a Child Guidance Clinic when she was eleven, suffering from severe phobic and hypochondriacal symptoms. She had a great fear and dislike of her body. When she grew up she had a phobia of lifts and trains, and was terrified of pregnancy. She was very shy and very flirtatious. She went into analysis in her late twenties, and she told me she gave her male analyst a hell of a time. The analysis was a success in so far as she got married and renounced her virginity, but the marriage deteriorated into violence and divorce. Louise then underwent professional training and developed her artistic talent in her spare time. She came into analysis with me after a crisis of depersonalisation in which she was frightened of going mad.

Louise was extremely anxious and controlling in sessions and had a bright, manic, false self. Her idealised positive transference hid fears of me as a sadistic controlling mother. She was able to work but was still restricted by phobias. Her father had died during her teens after a series of strokes which left him helpless and childish. Her mother had been concealing a breast cancer, which she revealed to Louise soon after therapy began. Louise helped nurse her mother and was rewarded by a change in her at the end of her life. From being a rigid clinging mother, she changed to an acceptance of her fate and real expression of love towards her daughters. Louise mourned her mother quite normally, I thought, except that she berated herself for not being continually in a state of deep depression.

Louise had compulsive thoughts which she thought were mad. If she did not button her shirt in a certain way her grandmother might go blind. She had violent impulses towards me while on the couch; for example, a sudden desire to take off her belt and hit me with it. She also had sudden loving impulses which upset her. She was terrified of her feminine feelings, which she described as 'slushy'. Her need for mothering distressed her because she thought it was homosexual. She had a false pride which made her hold out in a defiant way against what she called 'giving in'.

Fortunately, her painting was a way of helping her to accept herself as she really is, instead of having to be what mother approved of. She became aware of her identification with the creative activities of her father and grandfather. It took some time for her to accept the idea of her creativity as masculine. The first time I made an interpretation about a fellatio fantasy Louise could not accept what I said. A few minutes later she suddenly developed intense nausea and was frightened of vomiting. When she saw the connection the nausea subsided.

The analysis changed dramatically when Louise acquired a steady boyfriend called Patrick. She could no longer use me as a controlling disapproving mother, and she had to face the paranoid part of herself as a real obstacle for Patrick. There were several episodes of intense anxiety when she nearly wrecked her relationship with Patrick, but she came to see that her fear and anger belonged to her childhood. During this time she developed spots in front of her eyes with no organic basis, and also had herself investigated for breast cancer with negative result.

At the time of the session which follows, Louise had achieved some self-esteem but she still lived in a state of narcissistic omnipotence into which she retreated when threatened by anxiety. Patrick was slowly being transformed from an ideal object into a real person.

Louise began the session by saying she was feeling well in herself in spite of being worried about her blood pressure. She ruminated about which parent she is like in terms of the illness which she will die of. Will it be cancer or strokes? Then she said: 'I've stopped worrying about Patrick. It doesn't matter if he goes away for a few days, and I don't mind if he asks me to keep my distance. I can see he is frightened of being encroached upon. The squabbles at work don't bother me any more. I feel like learning again; I hope the feeling lasts. I've been looking at courses I might apply for. I have been thinking what a strange business analysis is, the way patients put things on to analysts. Clients do the same thing to social workers. But when you come to fetch me, I can see you are just an ordinary woman. At the same time I experience you as masculine.'

I said: 'You have escaped from the vicious circle of expecting to be put down every time you assert yourself, so you no longer experience your own powers as a threat to others. You don't feel you have to compete with me any more.'

Louise said: 'I have been thinking in a different way about how much longer I will need to come here.'

I said: 'Now that you have a continuing sense of yourself as a person to whom things happen, you don't have to feel you are in control all the time. You seem to be realising that what you put on to me in the transference can be taken back again.'

Louise said: 'Yes, I had a dream that I looked out of my window and the landscape was covered in snow. There was a pattern of gardens, not like it really is, with the gardens curving and interlacing. In my garden the snow had started to melt. It made me think of the Isle of Man with the Gulf stream keeping it warm. I remembered looking out the other day and seeing a man in a tree cutting off a branch. Then I remembered my father climbing a tree and cutting branches. I have only been able to remember him carrying that enormous plank of wood. It is as though he was ill so long I couldn't remember him when he was well. I was in a queue at the Post Office yesterday and a young mother was trying very hard to control her child without being punitive. There was a man in front of me who spoke to the child ... '. Here she broke down and cried.

There were three episodes of crying in this session: first, when she recognised me as a real person separate from the transference; second, grief at remembering her father in his prime; and third, about her mother. The scene in the Post Office revived a memory of her mother calmly resisting the manipulations of Louise's younger sister. She saw clearly that her mother had been identified with her own father as law-giver to the family in spite of the more usual recollection of family discord with mother putting father down. I commented on the difference between her present state of mind and her previous need to merge with her mother (or me) to avoid anxiety.

Louise said: 'When you said merge, I thought you were going to say murder.'

I said: 'That sums it up – if you merge, your separate identity is murdered.'

I have not tried to give a chronological account of the session. Instead I hope I have conveyed something of the way many different themes came together in an integrative experience.

– – –

I shall now refer to William Gillespie's paper, 'Woman and her Discontents' (Gillespie 1975), which is a masterly reassessment of Freud's views on female sexuality. Gillespie presents his conclusions in the form of questions which he prefers not to answer, thus providing an opportunity for others to do so. One question is a choice between rival theories. Does the girl who settles for femininity do so because she had given up the hopeless struggle to be a man, as Freud thought, or is femininity a primary condition which has to be abandoned for a time out of fear of the mother? Gillespie also asks whether Freud was mistaken in assuming that the clitoris is associated with masculine strivings. Could its excitement normally lead to the wish to be penetrated vaginally? In fact Gillespie wrote an earlier paper in which he discussed the finding of Masters and Johnson (Gillespie 1969). He showed clearly that the female genitalia function as a whole, and that the concept of vaginal orgasm is a myth. One can read that paper as a holistic description of female sexuality which supports my theory.

The approach I am advocating avoids the practical problems that a correct Freudian is still faced with. Nothing could be simpler than the indivisible wholeness of female sexual functions, once the idea of wholeness is used as a starting point instead of a phallocentric scientific view. Masculine striving associated with exclusively clitoral activity is a well known syndrome. The fact that such patients deny the existence of the vagina is eloquent proof that Freud was describing psychopathology and not ordinary femininity. The abandonment of sexual activity during latency is a cultural norm, but during these years the girl is still actively developing her identification with her mother. There is no slowing down of the interaction between mother and daughter, as persons or as part objects, which will determine the girl's adult attitude towards her body and her sexual behaviour. It seems to me that Payne answered these questions by adopting an integrative approach. The theoretical problems are the result of exclusively scientific thinking.

If we can develop a holistic understanding of male and female as complementary opposites which need to be integrated for healthy living, then perhaps some of women's discontent can be relieved, and competitive strivings replaced by freedom to take the male and female in oneself for granted. Gillespie writes about female sexuality as the dark continent. He also warns against going the way of Jung in saying that the penis stands for other less concrete things, rather than the other way round. Both these ideas are illuminated by thinking about feminine psychology as primary process. We have to acknowledge that Jungian thinking about the feminine provides universal concepts which are far more acceptable than Freud's view, which has caused so much confusion. After so many years of estrangement, perhaps a reconciliation will soon be possible. Reintegration of Freudian theory with Jungian knowledge of the feminine could produce a coherent theory of female sexuality. I think Sylvia Payne would approve.

4   The Pattern which Connects:[*]

A Review of *A New Science of Life*
by Rupert Sheldrake

Sheldrake's theory of formative causation is an evolutionary theory which explains those processes of growth and development which are not so far explicable by scientific knowledge. For example, it can be demonstrated that after rats in one laboratory have learned a new trick, similar rats in other places learn the same trick more quickly than they would have done before. When new chemical compounds are synthesised, it is often very difficult to get crystals to form. The more often a compound is made, the easier the crystallisation process becomes. Sheldrake's theory proposes the existence of a 'force' which he calls morphic resonance, which influences all natural processes in a non-energetic way. There are many gaps in our knowledge where it is usually assumed that scientific explanations will one day be found. Sheldrake's theory directs attention to those gaps in a new way which challenges the assumptions of science.

I have a lay person's interest in evolutionary theory and the history of ideas, which has grown out of the questions I ask myself as a psychoanalyst about how the mind works. My particular interest is in reformulating psychoanalysis in terms which are compatible with recent ideas in other disciplines. It seems to me a matter of some importance to find a new language for psychoanalysis which does not depend on detailed knowledge of how Freud's ideas have been developed. Although there is no direct connection, I believe that Sheldrake's work is part of a general trend towards holistic thinking which can

[*] First published in *Free Associations*, 1988, 11: 73–85.

contribute to the development of a unifying concept of mind. This will be discussed in the last part of this review. Before describing the contents of Sheldrake's book, I shall first sketch in the background of evolutionary theory from which his work has developed.

The book caused a furore when it was first published in 1981, because it expounds a hypothesis which seems to break all the rules of scientific investigation. The book was called 'an infuriating tract ... the best candidate for burning in many years' (*Nature*) and 'as far-reaching as Darwin's theory of evolution' (*Brain/Mind Bulletin*). Sheldrake's book assumes understanding of the concept of paradigm introduced by Thomas Kuhn in his book *The Structure of Scientific Revolutions* (Kuhn 1962). Kuhn's concept of paradigm, and in particular his concept of 'normal science', have changed the way people think about the development of scientific theories. A new theory is not simply the best available explanation. A revolution in science occurs when a new theory offers solutions to those problems for which answers have been urgently needed. The new theory is accepted because of its usefulness. It is not a case of one theory being right and the other wrong, although this may often seem to be so. In the excitement of new ideas, the limitations of a paradigm can be overlooked. It is because Sheldrake's ideas are outside the paradigm of 'normal science' that his book caused such a stir. The aim of this review is to suggest how his work might be significant for the emergence of a new paradigm for mind and mental illness.

There are always gaps in knowledge, which in theory does not bother scientists, but in practice the way people think seems to me rather different. An expert will not be bothered by gaps in his own field, because they provide a focus for his own questions. However, few people are expert in more than one or two areas, and we naturally assume that the current state of knowledge in other disciplines is 'right'. For example, I had always accepted that Darwin was right and Lamarck was wrong. I was interested to learn that Darwin tried to hold on to his belief in Lamarckism to the end of his life (Bateson 1980). Without detailed knowledge of the history of science, I find it difficult to imagine what it was like to learn about natural selection in the absence of genetic theory. Mendel's work was not generally known until after Darwin, and since it has been proved correct by countless experiments it is now integrated with later knowledge about heredity through the discovery of genes and then the cracking of the genetic code. Although Darwin's work has been combined with all this information, it is still only a theory which fails to explain many phenomena, and it is those unexplained areas that Sheldrake's work addresses. Lamarck's ideas were disproved, but have been given a new lease of life by Bateson, who approached the same information in a new way.

I have been describing the concept of paradigm with this illustration. Academic psychology is firmly fixed within the scientific paradigm and has to grapple with the problem of how to investigate subjective experience by means of an objective tool. As a psychoanalyst, I find it remarkable that conceptual frameworks are not usually discussed; analysts use Freud's instinct theory, and the various mutually contradictory object relations theories, without worrying about the implicit confusion of categories. Proposed changes in psychoanalytic theory are constantly made within this muddled context, while the wider issues are ignored.

The reception given to Sheldrake's book in 1981 followed the pattern Kuhn describes in his survey of the history of science. A new theory which upsets established knowledge produces violently conflicting reactions. Sheldrake was denounced as a charlatan by scientists convinced that there is no truth other than scientific truth, while others of broader outlook were prepared to consider the validity of his ideas. Sheldrake's theory challenges the orthodox mechanistic view of life that underlies all scientific activity, and in particular accepted views on evolution. The prevailing scientific view has been that all life processes can eventually be explained in terms of the known physical laws of matter. Psychoanalysts are involved in this paradigm to the extent that Freud's model of the mind was based directly on his expressed aim of creating a mechanistic theory of mind comparable to Helmholzian physics. Although we no longer talk about drives and energy in the way Freud did, the mechanistic basis of his theory remains intact.

At first acquaintance, Sheldrake's theory sounds like superstition or pseudo-science, because it offends against both

normal science and common sense. If one admits the possibility
that there is a non-energetic guiding principle involved in the
way organisms develop, then testing the theory becomes a
straightforward matter. Sheldrake was criticised for publishing a
theoretical book without experimental evidence to support his
theory. This deficiency was rectified when the second edition
appeared in 1985. The text was the same, but the book included
an appendix of the results of experiments carried out to test the
hypothesis, and reprints of some of the critical reviews of the
first edition. Sheldrake is a distinguished biologist, and his book
assembles evidence from published sources in a thoroughly
professional way. He does not say what morphic resonance is;
he deduces its existence from well known scientific evidence.
The tests were devised with suitable controls, and produced
statistically significant results which demand some other kind
of explanation if morphic resonance is deemed not to exist.
Those scientists who dismiss the whole hypothesis as rubbish
seem to have forgotten that such phenomena as electricity and
magnetism were investigated long before their true nature was
discovered.

A great deal is now known about DNA and the way in which
genetic information is transmitted. Enormous possibilities for
further research have been opened up by the cracking of the
genetic code. The work that can be done attracts a great deal of
attention. The gaps that exist in the network of information
attract much less attention. For example, the DNA available to
all four limb buds of a mammalian cmbryo is the same, yet they
regularly grow into arms or legs depending on their position.
Available knowledge does not permit the designing of experiments to discover how a limb bud is programmed to become an
arm rather than a leg. Sheldrake offers evidence that some other
force is at work, of a non-energetic kind, which he calls morphic
resonance.

The concept of morphic resonance challenges the usual
neo-Darwinian view that all evolutionary change is the result of
natural selection based on random mutations. It requires a
mental effort to shift oneself out of that state of mind in order to
get hold of the idea that morphic resonance, like a gravitational
field, is everywhere, and that the forms that develop are
influenced by a kind of blueprint due to the fact that such forms

have previously developed. It can seem mind-boggling that there is a different morphogenetic field influencing the development of each living thing, but if one thinks about it, the idea is no more unlikely than the diversity of life forms which actually exists.

Sheldrake is a modern representative of a rival school of thought which has been eclipsed during the past century but did not die out completely. The concept of morphogenetic fields, which Sheldrake has revived, was current in the nineteenth century among scientists who adhered to the theory of vitalism. Their views were not given credence because they were unable to produce hard evidence in support of their theory. In this century such writers as A.N. Whitehead (1925) and M. Polanyi (1958) objected to scientific materialism on philosophical grounds. Sheldrake's work is in direct descent from the ideas of C.H. Waddington, who formulated the idea of evolutionary pathways, which he called chreodes, in the 1920s (Waddington 1957).

Waddington used a model of a landscape made of sand to illustrate his concept of chreodes. The sand is grooved into branching paths which run downhill, so that if a ball is rolled down the slope, the path it follows is determined by gravity. Each ball that rolls down the slope will contribute to making one path well worn and more likely to be followed. The theory of morphic resonance that Sheldrake inherited from Waddington proposes that such channels become deeper through constant use, while 'unfavourable' channels are used decreasingly often. It is important to bear in mind the limitations of the mechanical model. It is only an analogy of the way morphogenetic fields are thought to influence the development of organisms, and the actual mechanism is not known.

Sheldrake uses an architectural analogy to emphasise the non-energetic nature of morphogenetic fields. In order to construct a house, bricks and other building materials are necessary. So are the builders who put the materials in place, and the architectural plan which determines the form of the house. The same builders, using the same materials and doing the same amount of work, could produce a house of different form by using a different plan. The plan can be regarded as a cause of the form of the house, although not the only cause. The house could never be realised without the materials or the activity of the builders. Similarly, a specific morphogenetic field is a cause of the form taken up by a system, although it cannot act without suitable building bricks and the energy to put them in place.

This analogy signifies that morphogenetic fields do not depend on conscious design, and that all causation need not be energetic, even though all processes of change involve energy. The plan of a house is not in itself a type of energy. Even when it is drawn on paper or realised in the form of a house, it does not have energy of its own. If the paper is burned or the house demolished, there is no measurable change in the amount of mass or energy; the plan simply vanishes. Likewise morphogenetic fields are not in themselves energetic, but they play a causal role in determining the form of the systems with which they are associated. For if a system were associated with a different morphogenetic field, it would develop differently.

Sheldrake starts from the orthodox neo-Darwinian position that the processes of random mutation and natural selection are themselves sufficient to account for purposiveness. Then he examines some outstanding problems in biology that have not been solved by that theory. Conventional biologists take the view that because science has explained so much already, they are justified in assuming that it is only a matter of time before the remaining gaps in the knowledge of the natural world will be filled in. Sheldrake focuses attention on these gaps, and by so doing draws attention to the limitations of the scientific paradigm.

The first unsolved problem concerns morphogenesis: how form comes into being. A bird's egg does not contain the structures that will be present in the newborn chick. Another mystery is the regulation of developing organisms. In the 1880s Driesch experimented with sea urchin embryos and showed that if one cell is removed at the two-cell stage, the remaining cell will give rise not to half a sea urchin but a smaller complete one. Conversely, when two embryos were made to fuse, one giant sea urchin developed.

Another unexplained mechanism is the ability of organisms to regenerate. The extreme regeneration of plants is rather taken for granted, but animals can also replace lost parts. If a flatworm is cut into several pieces, each piece will grow into a new individual. When the lens of a newt's eye was surgically removed, a new lens grew from the edge of the iris. This artificial regenerative process is more remarkable because the new lens grew from a different tissue than that of its normal origin in the embryo. Another extreme, if obvious, example of regeneration is the fact of reproduction. A detached part of the parent becomes a complete new individual. The conventional genetic explanation of these phenomena makes use of the computer analogy. It is said that the fertilised egg is programmed with DNA which specifies the organism's morphogenetic goals and controls its development towards them. It is not explained how the DNA, identical in each cell, is programmed to achieve different results in different cells. It is customary to say that this is the correct explanation because the paradigm requires that it should be so, but a moment's reflection reveals the enormous act of faith involved in that assumption. Sheldrake points out that the computer analogy leaves out the intentions of the programmer. In fact the mechanistic explanation, which uses such terms as 'goal directedness', ends up remarkably similar to the vitalist explanation.

Animal behaviour presents further challenges to the mechanistic theory. It is hard to imagine how DNA can account for the fact that young spiders spin webs without being taught. Young cuckoos who have been reared by foster parents congregate and migrate to join parents whom they have never seen. Animals 'know' how to regulate their own behaviour. Experimental animals continue to co-ordinate their movements even after their limbs or nervous systems have been seriously interfered with. A further problem which is usually passed over is that even if the nervous system of a simple animal could be understood so that the 'wiring' was known, we would still be unable to explain how the system came into being in the first place.

Sheldrake's work is revolutionary because he seems to have overcome the problem of lack of evidence that faced Waddington and the earlier vitalists. Waddington refrained from asserting that he was dealing with something outside the known range of physical causes, but there is no avoiding the fact that his concept of chreodes implies a guiding principle which includes the goal of development. Sheldrake has been able to bring the concept into the realm of falsification or verifiability by means of large-scale experiments.

The conflict aroused by Sheldrake's book is the latest round in an ancient controversy. Since the Enlightenment, the rise of science has favoured mechanistic explanations at the expense of vitalistic ones. Science seemed to have replaced the religious view of the unity of existence, in which all living things were part of the Great Chain of Being. Lamarck (Lamarck 1809) inverted the Great Chain by insisting that mind is immanent in all living creatures and can determine their transformation. He escaped from the negative directional premise that the perfect must precede the imperfect. He proposed an evolutionary theory which suggested a comparable unity working in the opposite direction. His work was eclipsed by the inexorable rise of science which determined that the appropriate paradigm for *The Origin of Species* was an attempt to exclude mind as an explanatory principle. I am indebted to Gregory Bateson's book *Mind and Nature* (Bateson 1979) for this information, and also for the fact that Darwin himself tried to hold on to his Lamarckian views until the end of his life.

Bateson is best known as one of the inventors of cybernetics and as the author of the double bind theory of schizophrenia. His concept of mind is an evolutionary theory which revives Lamarckian theory with a significant difference. Bateson attributes Lamarck's failure to a mistaken view of the nature of mind. Bateson's work is based on logical typing and information theory. It is interesting that Bateson mentions that his friend Conrad Waddington was contemptuous of conventional information theory, because it does not allow for the 'new information' generated at each stage of epigenesis (Bateson 1979: 57). Bateson's theory transcends natural selection with the idea that mind and evolution are stochastic processes; that is, they are goal-directed like the shooting of an arrow, but within the limits imposed by that directedness, the process is random.

Bateson quotes Alfred Russel Wallace, who seems to anticipate cybernetics in his recognition that natural selection is a conservative process:

> The action of this principle is exactly like that of the centrifugal governor of the steam engine, which checks and corrects any

irregularities almost before they become evident; and in like manner no unbalanced deficiency in the animal kingdom can ever reach any conspicuous magnitude, because it would make itself felt at the very first step, by rendering existence difficult and extinction almost sure to follow. (Wallace 1911)

Waddington wrote: 'An animal by its behaviour contributes in a most important way to the determining of the nature and intensity of the selection pressures which will be exerted upon it.' Bateson describes eight kinds of evidence that make the theory of natural selection untenable. He writes about behaviour and communication in terms of patterns of information which are ordered into categories by logical typing. If life processes are thought about in these terms – of information producing differences – it becomes obvious that any random mutation will rapidly be neutralised because it is an error in logical typing. For example, a more successful individual could destroy its own ecological niche by overgrazing; a short-term advantage becomes a long-term disaster.

The Lamarckian theory of the inheritance of acquired characteristics was disproved because learned behaviour cannot affect the DNA which is passed to the offspring. From the totally different viewpoint of formative causation, there is no essential difference between innate and learned behaviour, in that both depend on motor fields given by morphic resonance. In his discussion of Darwin and Lamarck, Bateson refers to the experiments of Conrad Waddington which form the background of Sheldrake's work. Bateson summarises his theory with the notion that the interaction of individual and environment proposes form; the genetic state disposes. With the idea that the unit of evolutionary change is the population, the whole picture changes. The individual has the capacity for adaptive change – that is, learning – but it is the population undergoing change by selective mortality that transmits the change to future generations. To quote Bateson again: 'The idea is now current that cultural inheritance is transmitted by making the infant receptive to the influences that are at work upon him.' In other words, the population as gene pool is subject to Lamarckian inheritance.

My interest in this subject began with David Bohm's theory of implicate order. In Chapter 2, I discussed the similarities between Bohm's ideas and Bateson's view of mind. The second edition of *A New Science of Life* (1985) contains a discussion between Bohm and Sheldrake of the connections between morphic resonance and Bohm's concept of implicate order. The two theories are highly compatible, and there is no difficulty about expressing morphic resonance in terms of implicate and explicate order. Morphic resonance can be thought of as one newly discovered aspect of the ultimate reality or holomovement, other parts of which have already been unfolded and made manifest in the explicate order of scientific reality.

Some critics of Sheldrake seem to overlook the fact that his theory does not replace science; scientific investigation is augmented by this additional point of view. What *is* threatened is the idea that scientific reality is all there is. Sheldrake does not write about psychology at all: his evidence comes from plant and animal studies, but nearly all the work that has derived from his book has been about testing human learning. After the book first appeared, simultaneous experiments were carried out on television in twenty-four countries. The idea was that if puzzle pictures were shown on television, with suitable controls, pictures that had been seen by many people would be solved faster in subsequent tests than pictures which had not been exposed. The results were statistically significant in Europe but, interestingly, much less conclusive in the US.

Sheldrake gives examples of the way human behaviour is influenced by cultural patterns. Although there is enormous diversity of behaviour and interests among human beings, the final goals of behaviour are relatively few. The perennial recurring interests of mankind do not vary. For example, the diverse cultural patterns of food gathering, food preparation and eating techniques all lead to the same process of chewing, swallowing and digesting. Similarly, diverse sexual behaviour leads to a consummatory act which is innate. If one uses Waddington's 'sand landscape model' to depict such behaviour, the picture is of a broad valley which becomes progressively steeper and narrower, ending in a canyon.

The psychological implications of morphic resonance have yet to be explored. There are obvious links with paranormal phenomena such as telepathy, precognition and synchronicity which are now subjects of serious scientific investigation. An

American organisation called the Tarrytown group offered prizes for the four most convincing proposals for testing Sheldrake's theory. In one of these Arden Mahlberg tested for the existence of collective memory by inventing a new form of the Morse code (Mahlberg 1987). Leaving out the letters S and O, the rest of the alphabet was arbitrarily assigned to new combinations of dots and dashes, suitably arranged to avoid unwanted side-effects. The results were as anticipated in that the Morse code was initially easier to learn, and that during the course of the tests the Novel code became progressively easier to learn. The results were taken to lend credibility to Jung's concepts of the archetype and the collective unconscious. The tests also showed that introverts were more influenced by the phenomena than extroverts, which is hardly surprising.

One can make a tentative attempt to apply Sheldrake's theory to psychoanalysis. Sheldrake's ideas fit rather well with Bateson's view of mind. If one accepts Bateson's notion that mind is immanent in all living things, then morphic resonance is an unconscious mental process. Sheldrake's theory includes inorganic processes which are usually excluded from definitions of mind. This problem exists only within the paradigm of normal science. In the theory of implicate order, scientific phenomena are aspects of the total reality which have been unfolded in the explicate order. In the ultimate reality or holomovement the difference between organic and inorganic, alive and dead, does not exist. Similarly, in systems theory all systems are parts of the whole. Jantsch (Jantsch 1980) states that every structure in nature is a sender and receiver of information.

In considering the possibility that morphic resonance is at work in the psychoanalytic process, one could start with the reinforcement of ideas in a patient's mind, both in terms of fixed patterns from the past and the effect of interpretations. The power neurotic ideas have in the mind, and the difficulty of dislodging them, could well be due in part to morphic resonance. The theory could also shed light on the reasons why therapy takes so long. Intense emotional experiences such as fear, anxiety or despair have been reinforced since childhood with the 'canyon quality' of Waddington's sand model.

The analyst could be influencing the patient through morphic resonance, which could reinforce the message conveyed by the consulting-room setting and the analyst's manner. It is possible, for example, that the tendency to regression could be reinforced by too-frequent sessions. Also, the patient picks up non-verbal messages which tell him about the analyst's philosophy of life and the countertransference. It makes a great deal of difference whether the analyst is a pessimistic scientist, a meliorist or a believer in primary envy. I suggest that such attitudes are conveyed as much by morphic resonance as by interpretations.

Sheldrake emphasises the distinction between the mechanistic theory of life and the metaphysical theory of materialism. If the mechanistic theory was to be replaced in biology by the hypothesis of formative causation (or any other theory) metaphysical materialism would still be a possibility, but it would have to compete with other metaphysical theories. After arguing the scientific basis of his theory, Sheldrake offers four alternative possibilities for its metaphysical significance. The first is a modified materialism, the second a conscious self not merely derived from matter. The third alternative is a creative universe in which a creative agency gives rise to new forms and patterns; this almost inevitably becomes a hierarchy of conscious selves. The fourth alternative is a transcendent reality which is the source of the universe and everything in it. This transcendent consciousness would not be striving towards some final form; it would be complete in itself.

Sheldrake's theory is one manifestation of a growing trend away from the traditional scientific world view towards a holistic mode of thinking. It is increasingly obvious that the paradigm of normal science is an inappropriate basis for psychoanalytical theory. I see Sheldrake's work as one aspect of a developing holistic view of mind which could lead to the possibility of integrating Freudian and Jungian theory, and other theories about psychotherapy, instead of the perpetuation and reinforcement of fragmentation and splitting that now exists.

To illustrate the way in which the wheel has come full circle, I can find no better way of ending than with the quotation from St Augustine which Gregory Bateson used as an epigraph to his book *Mind and Nature* (1979):

Plotinus the Platonist proves by means of the blossoms and leaves that from the Supreme God, whose beauty is invisible and ineffable, Providence reaches down to the things of earth here below. He points out that these frail and mortal objects could not be endowed with a beauty so immaculate and so exquisitely wrought, did they not issue from the Divinity which endlessly pervades with its invisible and unchanging beauty all things.

Mind and Nature is subtitled 'A Necessary Unity', and in the first chapter Bateson offers 'The Pattern which Connects' as an alternative title to the book. New theories will continue to increase our understanding of the pattern which connects. The pattern itself does not change.

5   Freud and Jung[*]

This paper has been adapted from a talk given to a small group of psychoanalysts in May 1990 with the aim of stimulating discussion about the relationship between psychoanalytic ideas and the changing intellectual climate in which we live. I have written several papers on the theme of the need to find a new paradigm for psychoanalysis in which I was influenced both by analysts who used ideas from outside psychoanalysis and also by the many holistic theories that have become popular in recent years. The point of a holistic theory is that it combines scientific and non-scientific ideas into a single world view. Science is not devalued, but it is placed in a wider context in which other viewpoints are not criticised for being non-scientific.

The concepts of primary and secondary process have undergone considerable change since they were first formulated by Freud. The name 'primary process' denotes that this is the kind of thinking we are born with – in which instincts and affects predominate – in contrast to 'secondary process', rational thinking which has to be learned. Dreams are the royal road to the unconscious because they are conscious manifestations of the primary process thinking which forms the boundless sea of the unconscious mind. However, Freud's aim of creating a science of the mind led him to overvalue rationality. The changes in thinking that have taken place since Freud have changed the way we see his work. The imaginative and intuitive aspects of his work are now more apparent than formerly, and we have more understanding of how small a part rational thinking plays in the lives of ordinary people.

[*] First published in *Free Associations*, 3(28): 642–54.

The basic theme in all this is the need to describe the change that has taken place in the way we think about the role of primary process. It is now more than thirty years since Charles Rycroft pointed out that psychoanalysis is a semantic theory, not a scientific one (Rycroft 1956). Many Independent Group analysts share this view, and yet the muddle of accepting supposedly scientific statements without demur continues. Bateson wrote that rigour and imagination are the two great contraries of mental life which need to be kept in balance (Bateson 1980). Bateson did not use the distinction between unconscious and conscious, but his way of describing the duality of the mind has considerable potential for linking psychoanalytic thought with other disciplines. In particular, this way of conceptualising the relationship of primary and secondary process is a development of Freud's original formulations, which makes it easier to speak about the use of imagination in scientific activity.

In addition it echoes Suzanne Langer's concept of discursive and non-discursive symbolism. Langer wrote:

> The great contribution of Freud to the philosophy of mind has been the realization that human behaviour is not only a food-getting strategy, but also a language; that every move is at the same time a gesture. (Langer 1942: 51)

She elaborated a thesis that the various 'impractical' apparently unbiological activities of man, such as religion, magic, art, dreaming and symptom formation, are basic human activities:

> The essential act of thought is symbolisation. We do not surpass animals in our perceptual skills but in our capacity to transfer perception into ideas. It is this capacity which accounts for those human traits which animals lack: ritual, art, laughter, weeping, speech, superstition and scientific genius. (Langer 1942: 43).

What follows can be attributed to the influence of these ideas on successive generations of the Independent Group, several of whom have written about symbolism.

This outlook is one in which scientific enquiry is seen as one aspect of the range of human activities, and cannot be separated from them in a general discussion of mind. I have become increasingly convinced that the so-called scientific attitude in psychoanalysis is a serious limitation. It is a mistake to think that science can explain everything in psychoanalysis, and it is a grave disservice to Freud to think that he was only a scientist. It was inevitable that Freud used the rigour of science as a basis for his theory; psychoanalysis could not have developed in any other way. In the cause of science Freud had to reject those of his followers who were insufficiently disciplined in their thinking. This was a great loss, particularly in the case of Jung. I have called this paper 'Freud and Jung' because I think that we are still suffering from the idea that Freud was right and Jung was wrong. I wouldn't want Jung without Freud, but I think many of his ideas are valuable, and complementary to Freud's.

It is my contention that analysts suffer from a kind of arrested development when they try to remain loyal to Freud's concept of science. In the same way that we can see the value of nineteenth-century scientific discoveries while knowing that knowledge has progressed since then, it should be possible to have a double vision of Freud's work, holding in mind both its amazing originality and its historical limitations. For example, it does not matter that Freud and Breuer used the reflex arc to demonstrate the mechanism of hysteria (Freud and Breuer 1893). We cannot see this as a valid scientific theory, but we can value the metaphorical significance of the attempt and the bold, imaginative leap that Freud made. My concern is that we do not have any conceptual framework for identifying those areas where Freud was actually wrong.

A holistic paradigm would make it unnecessary to label theories right and wrong, and would make it possible to accept and to integrate Jungian concepts instead of repudiating them. I have always felt sympathy for Jung because he stuck to his guns and refused to be intimidated by Freud, in spite of the great cost to himself. Jungians have an advantage over Freudians in that their basic theory is a holistic one, embracing myth and religion and cultural values. They can respond freely to the paradigm changes which are happening in the world, since they do not think of themselves as scientists. The other side of the coin is their lack of rigour; they borrow freely from psychoanalysis whenever they need to.

It seems to me that there is a historical irony, as well as a profound paradox, in the idea of psychoanalysis as a science. Freud's discoveries were about the irrational part of human nature, which is not amenable to science as usually understood; and furthermore, science does not admit of paradoxes. The idea that psychoanalytic investigation can lead to a scientific theory is fundamentally unscientific. Fortunately, this statement is also historically limited by the profound changes that have taken place in science this century. We tend to overlook the fact that Freud's science is completely outdated because the cause and effect outlook on life is still prevalent. Newtonian physics still provides satisfactory explanations for most of the phenomena of everyday life.

When particle physicists discovered that there are limits to certainty about the nature of matter, they turned to Zen Buddhism and other Eastern philosophies to find ways of describing their findings. The discoveries of relativity and quantum mechanics meant that the Newtonian universe ceased to be a valid metaphor. The holistic world view that preceded the Enlightenment in the West, and the cyclical world views of Eastern philosophy, took on a new relevance. These changes also give greater credibility to Jung's views, which were never confined by causality. It is now possible to think of science and religion as alternative metaphors for explaining the universe. George Trevelyan once said that the physicist's bubble chamber is the modern equivalent of the alembic of the alchemists, wherein man sees his own soul. The trouble with the concept of psychoanalysis as science is that it cannot address the primary importance of meaning. Papers written by Independents in recent years are increasingly concerned with this area. I shall discuss this in a general way and then give some examples.

The Jungian analyst Louis Zinkin wrote a paper about Bohm's work at the same time as mine (see Chapter 2), in which he demonstrated the harmony and compatibility of Bohm's holistic theory with Jung's psychology (Zinkin 1984). More recently I have read a book which spells out in detail the connection between implicate order and synchronicity. This book, by the physicist F. David Peat (Peat 1988), explores the myth of causality and shows that a great deal of faith is involved in our belief that cause and effect govern our lives. Even if we accept a reductionist scientific approach, we overlook the fact that cause and effect cannot be worked out in any detail. The number of variables affecting any given situation in life is so great and so unpredictable that there is no such thing as scientific certainty. It is more sensible, Peat argues, to begin with a holistic view which seeks meaning in the conjunctions and patterns of existence. Common-sense experience of cause and effect is only one limited way of understanding the world.

In any case, the insistence on scientific thinking contradicts a lot of what analysts actually do. Whatever our theoretical orientation we tend to agree that the totality of the experience of the session is of basic importance. I shall quote Anthony Storr on this point, from an essay on psychoanalysis and creativity:

> If Freud had been able to accept that play, fantasy and dreaming were attempts to come to terms with, and master, reality rather than to escape from it, he would not have had to lay down his arms before the problem of the creative artist, nor have felt that the grandest creations of art were unsolved riddles to his understanding ... Art and science are both concerned with seeking order in complexity and unity in diversity. (Storr 1985: 68)

In other words, Freud tried and failed to confine his theory to a scientific account of mental life, believing that fantasy had to be given up in the adaptation to external reality, whereas Jung was always aware of the value of the non-rational. There is plenty of evidence from Freud's letters and conversations that he did not succeed in convincing himself of the scientific nature of psychoanalysis. In terms of Bohm's theory, Freud equated reality with explicate order, while Jung was aware of the wider reality or implicate order. Scientifically minded people are guilty of a category error if they think that the value of psychoanalysis can be attributed to its status as a science.

As psychoanalysts we have a special insight into the inter-play of the rational and irrational in mental life, which can contribute to the evolving paradigm. The holistic view of mind as information implies that the way the mind works is ultimately the way the world is. The Western view of science and reality assumes cause and effect and linear time in a way that is unknown in other parts of the world. Freud seems to have been aware of this; for example, he suggested to Einstein, in their correspondence about war, that Einstein's physics was just as much a myth as his own theory (Freud 1933). It seems that the psychoanalytic movement, rather than Freud himself, created the myth that psychoanalysis is a mechanistic, reductionist science. In particular, it was Strachey's conscious intention, in translating Freud into English, to use the language of science. Despite the many virtues of the *Standard Edition*, the use of this text as the definitive version of Freud has meant that the imaginative and creative qualities of Freud's prose have been submerged (see also Freud 1933: 211).

Jung's insistence on the integrity of the personality and the search for wholeness is increasingly attractive as the times change. His interest in alchemy, once derided by rationalists, makes better sense in the context of the ending of scientific certainty. The idea of alchemy as bad chemistry did not hinder Jung in his understanding of the symbolism of psychic transformation. Furthermore, the notion of the collective unconscious is widely accepted outside psychoanalytic circles. Jung amassed evidence for the existence of recurring myths in different cultures, which demonstrate the workings of similar unconscious forces in different times and places. This cannot be proved scientifically, but it is absurd to disregard the manifestations of innate patterns of thinking because they are unscientific.

I will quote just one famous example (Jung 1927). When Jung was a young psychiatrist he saw a paranoid-schizophrenic patient squinting at the sun and moving his head from side to side. The patient told him the sun had a penis, which moved from side to side to create the wind. Four years later Jung came across an ancient Greek text about a Mithraic liturgy. It described a vision in which a tube was hanging from the disc of the sun. If the tube was to the east there would be a west wind; if the tube was in the west, an east wind would blow. Jung went on to point out that in some mediaeval paintings of the Immaculate Conception a tube reaches down from Heaven through which the Holy Ghost descended. The Holy Ghost was originally thought of as a rushing wind.

It was perfectly feasible to dismiss this kind of evidence forty or even twenty years ago, but nowadays it looks rather different. Heisenberg argued that ultimate reality is not to be found in electrons, mesons and protons but in something that lies beyond them, in abstract symmetries which manifest themselves in the material world, and which could be taken as the scientific descendants of Plato's forms. These symmetries can be thought of as having an immanent and formative role that is responsible for the material forms of nature. The concept of archetypal symmetries which can manifest themselves in the human mind is just one of many possible ways of stating this idea. (See Chapter 4.)

Theories are emerging from many different disciplines which treat mind and information as identical; I shall give two examples. The first is the new science of Chaos, which gives mathematical expression to the patterns of natural forms and events (Gleick 1987). Similar patterns, of unimaginable complexity, have been demonstrated in widely differing situations, from turbulence in liquids to the irregularity of coastlines, the unpredictability of the weather, and fluctuations in the stock markets. Fractal geometry, the mathematical basis of Chaos, has flourished with the development of computers, which can demonstrate how these patterns recur no matter how many times they are magnified.

The most striking example is the Mandelbrot set, which is illustrated in Gleick's book by a series of photographs of increasing magnification. From the beginning to the end of the series the magnification is x 1 million, with the same motifs repeating within each other on a smaller scale as the magnification increases. Each element in the pattern is part of the grand design, and at the same time there is a universe within each grain of sand which can be revealed by magnifying the pattern. Looking outwards, the single element could be said to represent the infinitesimal smallness of a human being in the cosmos. Looking inwards, it can be a representation of the infinite complexity of the human mind. My personal response to this book is to imagine that the patterns of Chaos could provide a way of describing the repetition compulsion. Compulsive behaviour follows a recognisable pattern, and yet each repetition is in a different context, from which it cannot be isolated. Is it possible that the rhythms of near-repetition in the patterns of Chaos could describe such behaviour? It is even possible that the study of these natural rhythms could reveal the innate patterns of mental activity.

The second example is the Gaia hypothesis, James Lovelock's concept of the world as a self-regulating organism (Lovelock 1982). Lovelock is an eclectic scientist and enormously creative. He has invented instruments to test his own and other people's theories, including some for space research. His theory is simultaneously scientific and holistic. Previous theories of life have held that plants and animals evolve on, and are distinct from, the earth as an inanimate planet. Lovelock has shown, through experiments of his own devising, that all living things are part of one great organism evolving over the span of geological time. This theory has provided a focus for many holistic ideas, particularly environmental ones. It points to the need for a new paradigm, and it is also compatible with Bohm's theory of implicate order.

I cannot mention Lovelock without touching on the psychology of creativity. Lovelock's immensely fertile mind is largely geared to solving practical problems, yet he must be using primary process to a large degree to conceptualise possible solutions. He exemplifies Sylvano Arieti's idea that we need the notion of a tertiary mental process to describe the successful combination of primary and secondary process in adults (Arieti 1976). This holistic concept would surely include the capacity to play with ideas (see Arieti 1976: 186).

If one accepts that there is an ordering intelligence informing the natural world, it follows that it is manifested in physical and psychological ways. Jung's concept of the collective unconscious is that it contains information which has never previously been conscious to the mind of the individual, in contrast to Freud's view. Now that the controversy between the two men is long dead, surely it is sensible to accept both theories.

The physicist Wolfgang Pauli, Jung's analysand and collaborator, was struck by the connection between psychology and physics. Jung and Pauli wrote that the physicist's investigation of matter and the psychologist's exploration of mind were different ways of approaching the same underlying reality (Jung and Pauli 1955). Perhaps mind and body are simply different aspects of a single reality viewed through different frames of reference (Storr 1987: 204).

Science changed, through quantum mechanics, from being impersonal to having to include the observer in the experiment.

Paradoxically, the supposedly personal nature of the mind was changed by Jung's work to include a deep impersonal layer. Meaning is the kernel both of material structures and the collective unconscious. This meaning is at the heart of the 'objective intelligence', that formative generative principle which is neither matter nor mind. This repeats Bateson's idea that mind is immanent in all living things. Bohm goes even further in his idea that everything is enfolded in the totality or holomovement, so that the distinction between animate and inanimate matter only exists in the explicate order of science and common sense. I find these ideas helpful in thinking about what really goes on in the process of psychoanalysis.

The progress of science produces ever-increasing specialisation and fragmentation which results in patterns of meaning being lost. This is a major problem in the world today which causes many people to reject science. In terms of yin and yang, Western society is heavily overloaded with masculine yang values. A holistic world view would restore the balance of masculine and feminine. Science does not address, let alone solve, the human problems of existence and it explicitly repudiates value judgements. In psychoanalysis this way of thinking has led to one of the worst muddles in the profession – the idea that anything less than five, or perhaps four, sessions per week is not proper analysis. The lack of consensus about the actual figure reveals its absurdity. This doctrine has persisted without regard to changing circumstances or the increasing length of treatment. We have ended up with a quantitative criterion of excellence, and no sign of a qualitative way of differentiating psychoanalysis from psychotherapy. This is the result of a supposedly value-free attitude; in practice it imposes hidden values on the patient. If patients are allowed to decide the frequency of their sessions, a more spontaneous and potentially creative situation is established. The same thinking applies to fees. If the patient participates in a discussion to agree the appropriate fee, many of the negative effects of an imposed fee and imposed rules can be avoided.

Now I shall give some examples of recent theoretical papers by members of the Independent Group which seem to me to be holistic in outlook. Perhaps the most important holistic thinker is Winnicott. His view of mental health as the capacity for illusion, the rejection of too much sanity, and the need for some non-integration, is a holistic and non-scientific view of analysis which has become implicit in Independent Group thinking. His concept of true and false self introduced a qualitative distinction between authentic and inauthentic behaviour which embodies Langer's belief that a meaningful existence is essential for mental health.

Nina Coltart's paper 'Slouching towards Bethlehem' was a personal statement of a holistic point of view which has been widely influential (Coltart 1985). In 1990 she gave a lecture on 'Attention' (Coltart 1990) in which she compared the quality of attention required of the analyst with the kind of attention that leads to enlightenment in Buddhist meditation. She quoted a passage by a Western Buddhist monk which could be taken without alteration as a description of the analytic attitude.

Dennis Duncan's paper 'The feel of the session' was about the quality of empathy (Duncan 1990). He has also written about the changing paradigm in the British Psychoanalytical Society. Michael Parsons explored the similarities of psychoanalytic technique and the martial arts of the Far East (Parsons 1984). He wrote of psychoanalysis as a way of being, and of the necessity for constant re-grounding in technique and basic principles in order to maintain this position. This paper illustrates in clinical terms a view earlier expressed by Karl Pribram:

> We need not polarize as opposites the hard-headed analysis and the search for structures (in the brain) and the wonder and awe when we view the embodiment of these structures. Those most productive of scientific fact have maintained, throughout a lifetime of contribution, just these spiritual qualities and as scientists they are ready and capable to defend spirit as data. This is science as it was originally conceived: the pursuit of understanding. (Pribram 1976)

In his appreciation of Marion Milner, Parsons summarises her work as follows:

> Her books are investigations of a state of mind which allows a deeper awareness of the truth precisely by giving up the assumptions of knowledge and opening one's vision as widely as possible to the unlooked-for and the unthought-of. (Parsons 1990: 423)

Another influential author who has no roots in science is Christopher Bollas. His work is concerned with the patient's individual idiom and the possibility of shaping one's own destiny through insight instead of being governed by blind fate (Bollas 1987, 1989). Although his approach is quite different, he has some similarities with Jung. I could mention many others, and there is no particular significance in my selection.

There is a vast difference between analysts with the outlook which I am calling holistic and those analysts who believe that psychoanalytic theory can be thought of as a set of scientific formulations. Analysts who think scientifically believe that everything is essentially knowable, an attitude which fosters self-aggrandisement. Perhaps it is the prerogative of the Independent Group to keep in mind just how little we know or can know.

I have used Jung as a symbol of a holistic world view which includes spiritual values. We need a comparable symbol for psychoanalysis to express the spiritual qualities in our understanding of Freud, which has been overshadowed by the idealisation of him as a scientist, and which has involved clinging to an outmoded concept of science. The change in attitude which I am advocating would answer many of the criticisms of psychoanalysis as unscientific. It is only with an outdated notion of science that psychoanalysis is devalued for not being something which it should not claim to be.

As the millennium approaches we can anticipate another psychological revolution comparable to the birth of psychoanalysis at the end of the last century. My hope is that as we witness the disintegration of the old order, the phoenix arising will take the form of a holistic paradigm.

6   Thoughts on the Healing Process*

This paper was first conceived as a talk to a small group of
London psychoanalysts who meet regularly to discuss new
ideas. My interest in holistic theories led me to consider the
psychoanalytic process in its entirety, and in particular the
relative absence of discussion of how it is that patients are
helped by therapy. After I had started writing, Vann Spruiell
published 'Deterministic Chaos and the Sciences of Complexity: Psychoanalysis in the Midst of a General Scientific Revolution' (Spruiell 1993). As far as I know he is the first psychoanalyst to make a comprehensive survey of the significance for
psychoanalysts of the revolution which has been taking place in
scientific thinking in recent years. He is particularly good on the
myths of science which need to be exploded and the liberating
effect this could have. He writes that

> if analysts pay attention to what they do within the analytic frame
> they will regain hope and a measure of freedom from the older
> constraints of obsolete and narrow conceptions of nature, e.g. 'the
> clockwork universe'. And it will be pleasant to no longer need to
> worry about whether psychoanalysis is a science. Instead we will
> ask in what ways does psychoanalysis fit in with other nonlinear
> dynamic systems? (Spruiell 1993: 33)

He suggests that although at present we can only use
deterministic chaos and fractals as metaphors, if psychoanalysis
can be seen as process the time will come when such models
can be made of psychoanalysis itself.

Spruiell discusses the work of American analysts who have

* First published in the *International Forum of Psychoanalysis*, 1993, 2: 149–54.

reformulated Freud in terms of systems theory. His general idea is that the structural model can also be thought of as a functional model, so that classical theory remains intact. Because Freud developed his theory from the results of his self-analysis, testing his perceptions and fantasies against rational observation, it is quite possible that he made a valid connection between the neurological and the psychological which could be brought up to date. I take a simpler holistic view, not being a Freud scholar, that psychoanalysis embraces the whole of human experience and can be linked with whatever is relevant to a particular context. Making computer models is one approach. Thinking about mental processes in ordinary human terms is just as important. Analysts have all along been practitioners of complexity theory, a colleague said to Spruiell. Many of the new ideas that analysts are writing about are concerned with interpersonal processes. We are undergoing our own paradigm shift away from the one-person psychology we have inherited. Some American analysts are returning to Freud's early formulations of the psychoanalytic process in preference to the structural theory. For example, Spruiell quotes Freud:

> I maintain that one should not make theories – they must fall into one's house as uninvited guests while one is occupied with the investigation of details. (Freud 1915b)

This suggests that Freud might well have had a theory of the collective unconscious if it had not conflicted with his scientific intentions.

Recently I heard a remark attributed to a Colombian Indian: 'Knowledge cuts up the world, wisdom makes it whole.' This has doubtless been said in other contexts, but it sums up what I have been trying to say and it makes a starting point for this exploration of my ideas about the healing process. I have been thinking how reticent we are in speaking about it. I think it is our private wisdom that we know about healing. It is much easier to share our knowledge of the techniques of analysis, and argue about them, than to discuss things which we experience intuitively in private, and which may well be damaged by exposure. It is wisdom and not knowledge that is the focus of this paper. Wisdom involves value judgements, knowledge does not.

Much has been written about the curative factors in analysis, and the literature about transference and counter-transference bears directly on this issue. Here I shall consider the subject from a different angle from the traditional medical and scientific models for psychoanalytic theory. I want to think about healing in a way that accepts the fact that many patients are helped by therapists and healers of all kinds. We may have the best techniques but we have no exclusive rights in this matter.

When we talk about transference we acknowledge that the process begins from the very first contact, and may often be present before that in the patient's mind. The likely success of a match between patient and analyst is based on a clinical judgement in which personal and intuitive factors play a large part. It seems to me that a patient's needs and wishes, hopes and fears make up a process of readiness to change. Anxiety and resistances can be left on one side for the moment. When I think about the most difficult patients I have seen, who stand out in my memory because they gave me the most trouble, they seem to have something in common. In spite of being very ill, or borderline, as we say, they all had a strong drive to engage in the treatment process. I interacted with them much better than I did with some less ill patients, a small minority of whom gave up treatment because they didn't know what they were looking for.

Now I will make a short diversion around the word 'borderline'. I used to think that the widespread use of this term indicated the inappropriateness of theoretical categories, that we were unable to devise a suitable classification because our theory was out of date. Since I gave up work in the National Health Service thirteen years ago, and with it the problem of filling in forms and labelling people, I have given up thinking about classifying people in that way. I now feel that although it is still unsatisfactory to place large numbers of people on the borderline between sanity and madness, the word itself may have value. As the traditional categories of scientific disciplines break down, most of the new ideas occur at the interfaces between established areas of knowledge.

To be on the edge, at a boundary, turns out to be of dynamic importance in many life processes. The sciences of complexity show that there is an oscillation, in both living and non-living systems, towards and away from states of total disorder. The boundary between one state and another is where things happen. One does not need to understand the mathematics to respond imaginatively to what is going on. The word 'border-line' acquires additional resonances if it implies an oscillation between two different states of being.

To return to the healing process. If patients can lock into therapy as if they know what they are after, it seems to me that they are behaving as if they had another chance to be a baby. The same idea was expressed by Daniel Stern:

> Certain categories of experience can never occur unless elicited and maintained by the actions of another, and would never exist as a part of known self-experience without another. (Stern 1985)

Patients invite us to provide in symbolic form the kind of experiences that they were denied the first time round. This might sound obvious but the change of emphasis is significant. It puts awareness of and response to what the patient is saying ahead of theoretical concepts of what the analysis ought to be about. It rules out an intellectual stance which assumes that the analyst knows what is best for the patient.

Consider, for example, the number of sessions per week. It has always seemed to me that the patient is the only person who can know the correct frequency of sessions. A certain amount of trial and error may be required, as with a nursing couple, but most babies settle to regular feeds. For the few patients who cannot express an opinion, building up from once a week is likely to provide a satisfactory answer. In every case a degree of flexibility is desirable; the patient should not feel under an obligation. Likewise both parties should agree that the fee is right. In this way a spontaneous relationship is entered upon, with boundaries maintained by the analyst and agreed by the patient. The way analysts are taught to manage their patients corresponds, in my view, to Winnicott's description of an infant forced into a compliant relationship with the mother (Winnicott 1971a).

I wonder about the process of change in analysis, and how it comes about that long-standing habits of thought and behaviour are abandoned as patients improve. The trauma or the fixation cannot be eradicated, but if analysis is successful somehow it doesn't matter any more; or at least it doesn't matter so much. We say the patient rediscovers a good internal object, or the bad internal object is expelled. How does this happen? The classical pattern of the progress of analysis is that after the defences are analysed, healthy development will begin. To put it another way, the patient has his or her personality taken apart and then he gets on with it. Formal descriptions of analysis sometimes sound like the patient being taken to the cleaners. I want to suggest that the transference relationship with the analyst as good parent engenders a healing process which exists in its own right. If we think about mental processes as analogous to physical processes, we can suppose that there is a natural healing tendency in the mind which corresponds to the healing of physical wounds. The separation of mind and body is an idea which is no longer tenable.

The process of healing can be brought about by other kinds of relationships than psychotherapy, and also by significant experiences, including religious ones. We may suppose that something equivalent to transference is frequently involved, and it may be that the process is largely self-engendered. I think the capacity for such experiences is closely connected with creativity, whatever that is. In any event we are looking at the replacement of abnormal mental patterns by healthy ones.

Now I shall describe a paradox of therapy which is quite easy to recognise. Clinical improvement can take place in the early stages of treatment while the analyst is still getting to know the patient. This can happen even if the analyst is feeling appalled by the range of pathology which is coming to light, which throws the original diagnosis into doubt. One can feel that the patient is much more disturbed than one first suspected, and still not have much of a clue as to what is going on in the transference, when suddenly there is a message that the patient is much better. The referring colleague may have heard that so-and-so is quite different since starting treatment, or the patient may report similar remarks made to him which he regards as nonsense. I have an unshakeable optimism which makes me believe that there *is* a healing process; and that like the transference, from which it cannot be separated, it starts from the very beginning. My theory about this is like two lines on a graph, with well-being increasing over time while the other line representing illness decreases. There are bound to be bumps and reversals, but it should be the case that a person who undergoes therapy derives benefit from it. My theory goes a little further. The second hypothesis is that a certain amount of progress towards being well is necessary before a patient can tolerate a painful truth which has been denied for years. This implies that some belief in oneself is necessary in order to work through depression.

Now I will explain what my optimism means in terms of the healing process. Pessimists may argue that I am indulging my patients' wish-fulfilling fantasies and analysis should be about disillusionment. I think my idea of healing means that the analyst takes the patient's wishes and desires seriously, because only if this happens will disillusionment result in a healthy person able to enjoy life in a realistic way, retaining the minimum of illusion that Winnicott tells us is necessary for healthy living.

This has implications for thinking about regression. Anxiety is often expressed about patients becoming totally regressed, as if this is an unavoidable feature of analysis. The model I have in mind explains how it is possible to work with early experiences and states of dependency without the patient losing the capacity to cope with adult life. What I am calling the healing process can be the capacity to tolerate states of mind relating to infancy because of feeling held in the transference relationship. Patients whose self-respect requires them to retain their autonomy are no less needy than those who cause anxiety by their capacity to regress.

There is a good example of this in Winnicott's paper 'Transitional Objects and Transitional Phenomena' (Winnicott 1971b). He describes a woman patient who relived symbolically the repeated loss of her mother through absences, including being lied to at the age of two. She was unable to make use of the rug, in spite of feeling cold, telling her analyst that 'reality is more important than comfort, and no rug can be more important than a rug'. Winnicott had refrained from offering the rug so that she could manage her own experience of loss. This patient was successful in keeping her adult life going between sessions and during breaks. I have always followed Winnicott's example and I have not had any difficulty with patients being unable to cope. There is a paradox about regression which I think I have taken from Winnicott, that successful temporary regression is a sign of ego strength, not weakness. The patient who refused the rug, and the artist who expresses primitive parts of his personality while painting, both rely on their own self-knowledge to undergo an experience which is worth having.

We hope that patients will come to see their past lives in a more realistic light. It is not just the accuracy or unconscious effect of our interpretations that produces insight. The giving up of defensive positions surely depends on feeling strong enough to give up psychological crutches. In the same way as a baby crying evokes a feeding response from the mother, I am suggesting that patient behaviour evokes a psychically nurturing response from the analyst.

The last part of this paper will be about an alternative way of thinking about the healing process. I shall be making a link between Winnicott and catastrophe theory, using a clinical example from outside psychoanalysis. Catastrophe theory is a fairly new mathematical method for describing the evolution of forms in nature. It was created by René Thom (Thom 1978) in his revolutionary book *Structural Stability and Morphogenesis*:

> It is particularly applicable where gradually changing forces produce sudden effects. We often call such effects catastrophes, because our intuition about the underlying continuity of the forces makes the very discontinuity of the effects so unexpected, and this has given rise to the name. The theory depends upon some new and deep theorems in the geometry of many dimensions, which classify the way that discontinuities can occur in terms of a few archetypal forms; Thom calls these the elementary catastrophes. The remarkable thing about the results is that although the proofs are sophisticated, the elementary catastrophes themselves are both surprising and relatively easy to understand, and can be profitably used by scientists who are not mathematicians. (Zeeman 1977)

Nothing could be further from Winnicott's work than computer sciences, and yet one of the characteristics of his thinking is his ability to find simplicity in apparently complex situations. I shall quote a familiar passage about the differentiation of inner from outer reality, where he writes about the intermediate area of experiencing:

> an area that is not challenged, because no claim is made on its behalf except that it shall exist as a resting place for the individual engaged on the perpetual human task of keeping inner and outer reality separate yet interrelated. (Winnicott, 1971b)

The process of oscillation between the inner and outer worlds is, I think, what enables us to value our intuitive insights as valid information about our patients. I shall consider the possibility that good and bad objects, or oscillation between states of trust and mistrust, could have physiological representation in the brain. Spruiell mentions a paper on catastrophe theory by Robert Galatzer-Levy (Galatzer-Levy 1978) which showed how this theory could add a qualitative dimension to psychoanalysis. Galatzer-Levy pointed out that psychoanalytic models ignore the relation of qualitative change to quantitative change. It is usually assumed that quality and quantity belong to different categories:

> Freud, A. Freud, Erikson, Mahler, among others, propose various epigenetic sequences. They ignore how the passage of time might result in qualitative change or imply that the observed psychological changes were the visible result of underlying biological changes beyond the scope of psychological investigation. Yet qualitatively new phenomena emerge as the individual develops. The predominant determinant of these changes is the passage of time. A qualitative change results from quantitative variation ... Analysts have dealt with the relation of qualitative and quantitative change in a variety of ways. The most common solution is to ignore the problem. For example, the use of the words 'overwhelm' or 'too much' in the discussion of trauma appears to continue quantitative discourse, but includes a reference both to quantity and resulting qualitative change. (Galatzer-Levy 1978)

Catastrophe theory was taken up in this country by the Oxford mathematician Christopher Zeeman. The summary of Thom's theory is taken from his book on the subject (Zeeman 1977). Since the mid-1970s Zeeman has been working on the applications of catastrophe theory to psychological phenomena, particularly anorexia and bulimia. He works with a therapist who makes use of the disturbances of consciousness in anorexics to induce states of trance. Apparently it is quite easy with a majority of these patients to induce trance and suggest that they can recover normal patterns of eating and sleeping. Patients are encouraged to develop the capacity for trance by themselves, which allows an escape from the terrors of the gorging and fasting so that they can think about their inner life. The eating compulsions and sleep disorder are thought to arise in the limbic system, and to represent the extremes of a pattern from which the normal middle range has been lost. All the features of the cyclical behaviour, apart from the original cause, can be described and predicted mathematically. The therapist believes that he does very little; Zeeman's description is reminiscent of those moments in analysis when an apparently trivial insight triggers off a complete reorganisation of the patient's inner life. Only patient and analyst know how much depended on that one moment. The event is random and unpredictable in its details and yet inevitable in its significance for the course of the analysis. I see this as an example of the analyst as practitioner of complexity theory. It seems worth noting in this connection that anorexia is one of the few psychological conditions in which it is possible to think about cure.

We have all heard the story about the patient who said to his analyst, 'Why didn't you say that before?', the point being that the analyst has been saying it for years. In the later stages of analysis I would think it is quite common for patients to have phases of insight alternating with loss of insight and repetition of old patterns of thinking. There is an alternation between two different states which can be experienced as being ill or being well. The impersonal analyst who refrains from directive interventions cannot influence the patient by suggestion or encouragement. If value judgements were to become respectable it would be possible to elicit the patient's co-operation and develop his confidence in his ability to get better. I suspect that many analysts do make subtle use of such techniques. It is not really possible to make interpretations without giving some indication of where they are leading. I can see no reason why this process should not be described and understood simultaneously in neuro-physiological and psychoanalytic terms. The model of the impersonal analyst may be as out of date as the concept of science which Freud used as a model for his theory of psychoanalysis.

I may seem to have demoted psychoanalysis by lumping it with all other healing processes. I want to redress the balance by asking again the familiar question, What is therapeutic in psychoanalysis? in the context of patients' general capacity for getting better. I find it hard to believe that our incredibly complicated theories are essential for interpretations to work. Here I shall misappropriate the well known lager advertisement. In the same way as ordinary beer can be good for you, ordinary therapies can also do good, but a good interpretation reaches the parts that other forms of therapy cannot reach.

Insight brings the possibility of symbolic transformation of infantile experiences. The patient can then think freely and with understanding about traumatic events which were previously inaccessible and being experienced concretely. It is the innate capacity to understand symbolic meanings that determines whether patients will respond to therapy or not. This cuts across ordinary classifications of kind and degree of psychopathology. Some people seem to be able to use therapy without any apparent self-awareness. I like the idea that these events happen in the limbic system. Could this be the part of the person that we know how to reach?

Surely it is to our disadvantage to remain isolated from the enormous amount of information about mental processes coming from neuroscientists. Karl Pribram wrote:

> The potential energy between mind and matter appears to lie at the interface between matter and meaning, where a physical signal in the brain becomes an experience in the human mind. (Pribram 1989)

We could all write volumes about our experience of change in patients, each of us using a more or less private psychoanalytic language which would be understood by some and repudiated by other members of our society. If we pay attention to the changes in thinking produced by investigators in other fields, we might develop a language that would be recognisable to large numbers of people, instead of proliferating abstruse theories within our divided society. For example, it might be possible to link catastrophe theory with Matte Blanco's work on infinite experiences.

A final thought about wholeness and healing. As I have indicated at several points, the scientific process fragments knowledge, and our theory is seriously lacking in concepts of integration and healing. This has reflected the state of affairs in the world over the past forty years. Hopefully the recent proliferation of holistic theories will soon be reflected within psychoanalysis. From this perspective loyal adherence to Freud or Klein is just as counterproductive as the loyalty of damaged children to their parents. In both cases pathological attachments are formed which interfere with healthy functioning. Unless we can take part in the changes that are going on in other areas of thought, psychoanalysis will be increasingly marginalised. Even if Spruiell does not inspire analysts to study computer sciences, his paper will have an important effect because he speaks authoritatively about Freud. I am trying to do the same thing on the limited basis of my individual understanding. It is not necessary to follow the mathematics to see where these new ideas are leading us, because the patterns of nature and the patterns of mind can resonate directly for anyone who can relate to them. We use our innate knowledge in every theory we construct, however personal or trivial. We are aware of the fragility of our individual experience. It is a source of inspiration and excitement to find that one's private metaphors occur elsewhere.

7 Dreamwork Beyond Psychoanalysis*

This paper discusses the healing process in dreams which has been developed by Dr Montague Ullman in the dream groups which he started in the 1970s. After an account of my participation in a dream group, there follows a discussion of the ideas which influenced him and some comments on the significance of his work for psychoanalysts. Dr Ullman is always known as 'Monte' so I shall use that name for him.

Monte was born in New York in 1916 and trained there as a doctor. He specialised in both neurology and psychiatry, and in addition he was involved in research into extra-sensory perception. This began with some remarkable experiences in telekinesis with a group of friends when he was a medical student. He practised as a psychiatrist and psychoanalyst, and he also founded a dream laboratory at the Maimonides Medical Centre. There he was in charge, throughout the 1960s, of a prolonged investigation into dream telepathy, about which he has written extensively (Ullman et al. 1973). He is now Emeritus Clinical Professor of Psychiatry at the Albert Einstein College of Medicine. In 1976 he gave up his psychoanalytic practice and went to Gothenburg for a year to teach psychodynamic psychotherapy to psychologists. His course on working with dreams attracted the attention of psychoanalysts and psychiatrists in Stockholm, so that a seminar group was formed. From this beginning the first dream groups consisted of mental health professionals, but soon included anyone interested in dreams. Later on, groups were started in many different contexts such as schools, families, art centres and community groups (Ullman and Zimmerman 1979). All these groups were set up on a basis of equality, using

* First published in the *International Forum of Psychoanalysis*, 1995, 4: 91–5.

a technique which differs significantly from psychodynamic group therapy as we know it.

Monte's approach to dreams had several roots. He had been listening to patients' dreams for many years and was interested in the social referents that they so often contain. He had long been aware of the metaphorical significance of dreams and did not find psychoanalytic theory helpful. He wrote of his method that it was 'as if each dream was the dreamer's own on-target theory of his or her existence at the moment'. The skills he used were to listen to the unique life experience that resulted in that particular theory, and to talk to the patient in a way that made it possible to transform the theory into living experience. His awareness of the sociological dimensions of dreams made him realise the relevance of the work of Trigant Burrow, who had been an influence on Foulkes in the development of group psychotherapy (Burrow 1973).

Monte's year in Gothenburg turned into eighteen months, followed by extended twice-yearly visits to Sweden. There is now a national society for the study of dreams in Sweden with groups in most major towns. I shall describe his method in his own words. There are five underlying premises and three principles.

First premise. Dreams are intra-psychic communications that reveal in metaphorical form certain truths about the life of the dreamer, truths that can be made available to the dreamer awake.

Second premise. If we are fortunate enough to recall a dream we are then ready, at some level, to be confronted by the information in the dream. This is true regardless of whether or not we choose to do so.

Third. If the confrontation is allowed to occur in a proper manner the effect is one of healing. The dreamer comes into contact with a part of the self that has not been explicitly acknowledged before. There has been movement towards wholeness.

Fourth. Although the dream is a very private communication it requires a social context for its fullest realisation. That is not to say that helpful work cannot be done by an individual working alone, but rather that a supportive social context is a more powerful instrument for the type of healing that can occur through dream work.

Fifth. Dreams can and should be universally accessible. There are skills that can be identified, shared and developed in anyone with sufficient interest. Dream work can be effectively extended beyond the confines of the consulting room to the public at large.

It bears emphasising that dreams are intra-psychic communications. The process I use is geared to the needs of the dreamer as the one to whom the dream is being communicated. Communication to the group is a secondary affair necessary only for the group to make its contribution to clarifying the dream. So three principles can be stated:

1. respect for the privacy of the dreamer. Each stage of the process is designed to be non-intrusive so that the group follows rather than leads the dreamer. The dreamer controls the process and there is no pressure to go beyond the level of self-disclosure which feels comfortable.

2. respect for the authority of the dreamer over his or her dream.

3. respect for the uniqueness of the individual. (Ullman 1993)

Now I shall describe the procedure used in Monte's dream groups. A group meets once or twice a week, or less often. Once a group is established, leadership rotates between the members. At each session someone volunteers to present a dream. If more than one person does so, precedence is decided either by discussion between them or by tossing a coin. The dreamer then tells the dream, perhaps from a written record, repeating it slowly so that everyone can write it down accurately. The second stage belongs to the group. Members first describe their feelings about the dream, using the first person, and then move on to offering metaphorical insights in the same way. The use of the first person makes it clear that contributions by the group are projections which can be used or disregarded by the dreamer, the group having its own experience at the same time. Questions may be asked, to elucidate details or suggest a particular focus, but the dreamer is always in charge. The dreamer then responds to the group by telling of the associations evoked by the discussion. There follows a dialogue between the dreamer and the group, which begins with a search for contextual clues. Then there is a playback, with one member reading back to the dreamer the original account of the dream, one scene at a time. The dreamer responds with reactions and associations. After what has gone before, this can be a highly charged experience for all. There follows an orchestrating stage in which insights are offered. A final stage can be the dreamer presenting additional comments at the next meeting of the group.

I went to Stockholm in October 1994 to attend a weekend workshop. There were people in the group from all parts of Sweden, many of whom had worked with Monte for a long period and then gone on to run their own groups. Because I had been corresponding with Monte for some months I was not intimidated by the prospect of joining in with experienced dreamers, but of course I did not know what to expect. The language used was English, and the dreams were read out in Swedish as well. It was an emotional occasion because Monte had not visited Sweden for two and a half years, but at the same time many of those present had not met each other before. I felt welcomed and valued. This group met only a few days after the Baltic ferry disaster, and the first session was quite sombre. At first the atmosphere was rather flat and I found the procedure mildly irritating, because it is so different from the therapeutic process I am used to. However, by the end of the session I had cottoned on to the fact that interpretation is out. At several points, Monte, who was leading the group, stopped somebody asking a question and made them reformulate it as a suggestion. When the second session began on the next day, I felt I had become part of the process. As the weekend proceeded the level of intensity rose and the last few presentations were remarkable.

That workshop led me to explore the influence on Monte of the work of Trigant Burrow, which I had not encountered before. Burrow was born in Virginia in 1875 and was, from all accounts, a very impressive and talented person. He trained as a doctor and psychologist and became the first American-born psychoanalyst. He met Freud and Jung in New York in 1909 and spent a year in Zurich in analysis with Jung. He was a founder of the American Psychoanalytic Association, and its President from 1925 to 1926. He corresponded with Freud for many years and also with Jung, but he diverged from psycho-analytic thinking because of his emphasis on the social nature of symptoms. He had an idea which seems fairly ordinary now, but was unacceptable at the time – that it is society that is sick and not the individual. He set up therapeutic groups and then a therapeutic community, insisting on the equality of members and leader. Burrow was the first to use the term 'group analysis'. He later renamed his own work phyloanalysis, which left Foulkes free to use it.

In 1919 Burrow described a primary subjective phase of life in which the infant is identified with the mother. He called this a nesting instinct. He realised, unlike his contemporaries, that neurasthenia and psychosis have similar causes. He believed that the harmony and connectedness that exist between mother and infant should also exist between the individual and society. He realised that so-called normal behaviour is not at all the same thing as mental health. As a result of his interest in the new physics he thought of consciousness as one mass, out of which the individual develops, and so he found the current technique of psychoanalysis too narrow a focus (Burrow 1973).

Burrow wrote that the community occupies the same position within the social unconscious as the mother image does within the individual unconscious. He saw this idea as a natural extension of psychoanalysis to the social sphere. In 1925, when relativity and quantum theory were relatively new, Burrow wrote that Freud's static ideas were like Newtonian physics compared with his own dynamics. I find it interesting that fifty years later I was making the same point in putting forward David Bohm's theory as a better model of the mind than Freud's attempt at a scientific theory (see Chapter 2). Bohm's theory of implicate order, based on quantum physics, does away with the duality of mind and matter. Burrow's language is very dated but clearly he took a similar holistic view. A holistic view of psychoanalysis, that is, seeing it in the context of all the rest of the world, throws into relief the narrowness of outlook of those people for whom the whole world is viewed through psychoanalysis. The point I am making is that in addition to focusing on the view from the patient's inner world we can and should see things the other way round. It is often the acquiring of this ability through therapy which enables patients to recover.

In this connection I think it is significant that Monte thinks of himself as a teacher, not an analyst. In my paper on healing (Chapter 6), I drew attention to the relative lack of interest in the process of how patients get better. Surely a significant part of what we do is enabling the patient to learn and grow, which is educational rather than analytical.

My experience of the dream group in Stockholm stimulated many thoughts about the nature of the transference and how we use it. There is a delicate balance between interpreting in the transference and being present for the patient as oneself. I have suggested that the usual ways of describing the analytic situation do not take into account the healing process as a natural tendency. The essential requirement for healing to occur is the establishment of trust. Monte gave up working as a psychoanalyst because formal analysis could not provide a framework for the work he wanted to do. The method he developed for dream groups is totally non-intrusive. In particular, by requiring the group to use the first person in the initial stages of the discussion, confrontations are avoided. I find this an interesting challenge to our technique of interpretation, which has been handed down as essential to the scientific nature of the analytic enquiry. Following Burrow, Monte takes the view that the detritus of a sick society clutters up our dreams. Through alienation, and centuries of rationalism, we are out of touch with the capacity to understand dreams which some societies have enjoyed since biblical times.

There is evidence from recent studies of child development, and many other sources, of the infant's need for an environment of trust from which the outer world can be safely explored. Colwyn Trevarthen has introduced the concept of companionship as one of the activities of the newborn (Trevarthen 1994). He describes a process which can be observed a few hours after birth, of actively engaging with another person by imitating their actions and expressions. This seems very like a new version of Burrow's idea of social instinct.

I am writing about groups without any direct experience. I

do not want to compare dream groups with group analysis. Monte's dream groups are a more direct reflection of Trigant Burrow's ideas, because of the emphasis on equality and the elimination of transference. I have been impressed by the similarity of Monte's thinking about dreams to Rycroft's approach. In his book *The Innocence of Dreams* (Rycroft 1979), Rycroft takes the view that dreams express the biological destiny of the dreamer, in that they represent a commentary on the important circumstances of life; birth, reproduction and death. It is a small step from this idea to the inclusion of social relating as part of biological destiny.

Rycroft's book has an implicit meaning which has not, as far as I know, been generally recognised. While giving Freud a central place in the history of dream interpretation, Rycroft argues that the distinction between manifest and latent content and the insistence on free association are unnecessary. I think this means that although Freud recognised that dreams are the royal road to the unconscious, more recent developments in psychoanalysis have not fulfilled the promise of his discovery. Analysts' reports of their interpretations of patients' dreams can sound as if they are made on the basis of the analyst's theoretical position rather than a true understanding of why this person has this dream now. Monte's dream groups are evidence of how dreams can help people to understand their own lives. Monte points out that the obvious psychoanalytic interpretation of the symbols in a dream often differs from its current significance. The true meaning can only be discovered by the dreamer, the group assisting in the process.

Monte has updated Trigant Burrow's idea of innate species connectedness by showing how it can be discovered through dreams. People who work together in a dream group develop a sense of trust and solidarity. The innate honesty of dreams helps people to understand their predicaments and in doing so to respect their own inner nature. Monte knew David Bohm and his work for many years, and he sees dream life as the closest we can get to awareness of the implicate order of reality which underlies the world of appearances. There is also a close connection with Jung's concept of the collective unconscious. Freud wrote in his paper 'The Unconscious':

It is a very remarkable thing that the Ucs of one human being can react upon that of another, without passing through the Cs. This deserves closer investigation. (Freud 1915a: 194)

Unfortunately he does not seem to have followed this up, but we do know that towards the end of his life he was much more accepting of the possibility of genuine paranormal phenomena; that is, of communication between people by other means than consciousness. Jung wrote that we are dreaming twenty-four hours a day but we only become aware of our dreams when conscious thinking ceases. Burrow extended Jung's ideas with his own concept of a collective social unconscious. He believed that the individual is forced to adapt to the socially conditioned pattern of what is right and wrong. This seems to anticipate Winnicott's work on the true and false self. Burrow believed that society demands that the individual betray his basic nature in a way that is ultimately a threat to the survival of the species. He understood that we all need to learn to live together in society in the way that animals live together in social groups. There is now abundant evidence from ethology of the social life of animals which was not available to Burrow, of an innate biological need to belong to a group.

Monte built on these ideas of Burrow's with his belief that dreams provide us with honest reflections of ourselves. This prompts me to think about the relationship between inner and outer reality in our work. For many years I held on to my belief in the necessity of working in the transference by telling myself that only in this way can the symbolic meaning of symptoms and behaviour be conveyed to the patient. However, like many others, I have given myself permission not to make transference interpretations whenever it seemed to me that the patient was not ready to accept them. I have also seen that strict adherence to orthodox teaching can produce situations where the analyst abuses the power he or she has over the patient. For example, the refusal to answer questions can be deeply wounding and also an offence against ordinary courtesy. Here the question of trust comes up again. One can retain a patient's trust by explaining sympathetically why asking questions is inappropriate, but silence or refusing to explain will induce mistrust. It is very striking how little agreement there is, after a hundred years of psychoanalysis, about what is effective in treatment.

It seems worth speculating on why this is so. Freud took social values for granted in a society where conformity was the rule. Nowadays society has fragmented so much that the very idea of a standard of behaviour worthy of general acceptance is difficult to formulate. Freud's idea of the analyst as impartial observer has been rendered obsolete by decades of work on countertransference, but authoritarianism still prevails in the attitude students are taught to take with patients.

Taking part in a dream group made me question the basis of the psychoanalytic procedure. It made sense when analysis lasted a matter of months and when the idea of analysis as a scientific enquiry made sense, to provide a laboratory-like setting in which the patient's drama could be played out, understood and resolved. We are now in a completely different situation. Many patients do not have the usual Oedipal experiences, treatment continues indefinitely and often lacks a clear goal. We no longer have the expectation which enabled Freud to call his method psychoanalysis. Our patients quite often know all about themselves; it is meaning that escapes them. The formal method, rigidly applied, can encourage resistance and regression. Excessive interpretation in the transference can also delay healing by obscuring the possibility of the patient being in charge of his or her own life.

The problem for analysts has always been that we are trying to describe the irrational in rational terms. Dreams represent the basic stuff of the mind out of which rational thinking develops. It makes sense to focus on the problems of the individual in order to understand them, but it seems increasingly important to consider the interpersonal when thinking about a person's life as a functional whole. In his recent book *The Age of Extremes*, Eric Hobsbawm wrote:

The cultural revolution of the later twentieth century can ... be understood as the triumph of the individual over society, or rather, the breaking of the threads which in the past had woven people into social textures. (Hobsbawm 1994)

Monte's dream groups offer a remarkable opportunity for ordinary people to rediscover their capacity for healthy interaction with others, at the same time as they gain insight into their own inner life. This suggests to me that new social textures might be woven by rediscovering ancient ones through dreams.

8   Dreams, Imagination and the Self*

Now that psychoanalysis is a hundred years old we can look back to explore the sources of Freud's creativity. When Freud was a young man he was a passionate admirer of Goethe and used him as a role model. Goethe was born in 1749 and died in 1832, twenty-seven years before Freud was born. His long life spans the vital phase when modern science and the modern mind were young and growing vigorously. Before the end of the eighteenth century he was already famous for his achievements as a poet, novelist and dramatist, but above all as a fully realised personality T.J. Reed describes Goethe's life and work as monumentally normal beside many of the developments in literature and men's thinking about literature since his time:

> [T]he growing existential gloom; social marginality of writers; the 'poètes maudits', with their deliberate deranging of the senses; the pursuers of art for its own question-begging sake; the hermetically obscure, the agonisers over how to write at all, the despairers of ever conveying thought; and most recently the dehumanisers of literature who would detach it from its roots in life and make it a self-referential game, sabotaging men's most valuable form of open communication by simplistic doubts of its viability. Beside all this, Goethe's normality is not antiquated but defiant and invigorating. He stands high above this subsequent modernity ... luminous against the dark. (Reed 1984: 101–2)

I shall use this image of Goethe two hundred years ago, and the birth of psychoanalysis a century later, to look at the development of the self.

* This is the text of a lecture which formed part of a day of public lectures called 'What is the Self?' at the Institute of Psychoanalysis on 1 February 1997.

The history of the self is inseparable from the evolution of consciousness. Before the Enlightenment religion was the chief source of knowledge about the world. Within the accepted framework people knew their place in what was felt to be the natural order of things. Man was seen as the pinnacle of God's creation, a microcosm of the macrocosm. The world was the centre of the universe. Man was linked through invisible connections to the rest of creation by what has since been called, in Lovejoy's famous phrase, the Great Chain of Being (Lovejoy 1936). There was no concept of evolution or progress; mans' task was to redeem his fallen state, which was viewed as a temporary separation from the unity of the spiritual world which would be ended by death.

The astronomical discoveries of Copernicus and Kepler turned the mediaeval world inside out by showing that the earth moved round the sun. Descartes caused an equivalent philosophical revolution when he separated the thinking self from the external world. He began by doubting everything, and came to see truth as that which can be clearly and distinctly conceived. From the existence of the doubting and imperfect subject, himself, Descartes deduced the necessary existence of a perfect God. Only an omnipotent God could account for the reliability of human reason and the objective reality of the phenomenal world. In his view everything man perceives is external to himself. The cognitive capacity of human reason and the objective reality of the natural world had a common origin in God.

This separation formed the basis of scientific objectivity. Henceforth the world was to be explained in terms of cause and effect. This was the beginning of self-conscious awareness, and the use of the word 'ego' as a noun and the word 'consciousness' date from this time. The centre of gravity of human thought shifted from the cosmos to the mind of the individual. The ideas and emotions a person experienced were now his own property and no longer the result of external agencies or divine influence.

This meant that concepts of morality shifted from the world of action into the inner world of the individual. Strength of purpose, self-control and generosity of spirit became the ultimate virtues, and were used in the domination of passion by thought. The way in which men exercised their free will was the test of virtue; generosity was inseparable from dignity or self-esteem. This new moral order under-pinned the achievements of science. It is often overlooked that the early scientists were devoutly religious; in the early stages scientific discoveries seemed to clarify the claims of religion. It was only much later that the moral basis of science was abandoned in the formation of the modern outlook. What started as scientific method became the only way of looking at life. By this process of separating the thinker from the thing observed, meaning has been progres-sively lost from the material world. This is the profound difference between our scientific age and the previous one, when meaning flowed through all things and connected them.

Goethe is significant because while he inherited the old order, he belonged also to the modern world. He was part of the decline in traditional beliefs which forced every thinker to see the world with new eyes. He was also part of the new scientific age which reached its full flower during his lifetime. He pursued his own scientific investigations throughout his life. He is a symbol for psychoanalysis because he realised that the natural world, of which we are part, is the basis of our existence. He thought that our perception of ourselves as part of nature is what makes us value life. Goethe did not think he was discovering new facts, rather that he was opening up a new point of view. He realised that the scientific method was not the only possible one; he said scientists should be trained to observe qualities. While his contemporaries were detailing the structure of the different parts of plants, Goethe was concerned about the relationship between the parts. Through imaginative contem-plation of the outward forms he came to understand the activity producing them; his theory of metamorphosis translates the nature of the plant into an idea of the plant in the mind. The plant is not viewed as an inanimate thing, it is seen as something alive, evolving and becoming. The whole universe is experienced as living and growing. In these ideas Goethe carried forward the mediaeval tradition of holistic thought. In contrast to Descartes' famous statement 'I think, therefore I am,' Goethe wrote 'I was dreaming and loving as clear as day; I realised that I am alive' (Goethe 1964: 285).

Goethe took the view that man is more likely to notice what he lacks than what he possesses, and concentrating on what he lacks inevitably produces a shrinkage. This in itself could be a metaphor for psychoanalysis; it is often the very thing that a patient cannot see when he or she seeks treatment, and can see at the end of it. Several of my patients have referred to this change as joining the human race. Goethe's view anticipates modern jokes about shrinks, which depend on unconscious recognition of people's reluctance to give up their attachment to childish or envious behaviour.

Freud's passion for Goethe is for me a symbol of his imaginative capacities which could not be confined by the science of his time. A powerful romantic undercurrent flows through Freud's thinking, which he often expressed in quotations from Goethe's works. He was particularly fond of quoting from Faust; this occurs strikingly often in 'The Interpretation of Dreams'. Freud took from Goethe a holistic spiritual world view, which has been overlooked for many years but is now relevant again in the light of recent developments in science, which I will come to presently. For Goethe, art and nature followed the same laws. He saw in great works of art an essential truth which he experienced as identical with the workings of nature revealed by science. He paraphrased Plotinus, the third-century Neoplatonist, as follows:

If the eye were not sun-like, it could not see the sun; if we did not carry within us the very power of the god, how would anything god-like delight us? (Goethe 1964: 282)

Goethe's own scientific observations were inseparable from his interest in art, and he thought that humans fulfil their potential in the same way as a flower unfolds. He realised that the human mind plays a constructive role in all knowledge; therefore he rejected the dualism of science. Rather than seeing man imposing order on nature, he saw nature as permeating everything. He did not see spirit as separate from nature, rather that nature is itself spirit. He wrote that the states which scientists observed were inappropriate, because in life nothing stands still and everything is motion. Within the controlling framework of scientific rigour, Freud's writing, like Goethe's, is extremely vigorous and creative. I want to show that Goethe's influence is central in Freud's work.

Scientific investigation has been a very powerful tool which has changed the material world enormously. We now enjoy the benefits and we take them for granted. It has become a widespread belief that scientific truth is the only kind of truth. The world of appearances, that which can be viewed objectively, is mistaken for the real world. As this process has continued over the past two centuries it has had the effect that people increasingly see only the appearances, or the rational. Anything that does not seem to be in accordance with the objective world ceases to have any meaning. It is not realised that this is a learned way of seeing the world, particular to our culture. By this process of alienation people are more and more cut off from the natural world and from its manifestation in their own nature.

This disintegration of the self is expressed in twentieth-century literature as the impossibility of self-knowledge or security of conviction. At the same time the search for self-knowledge is felt to be all important. There is no alternative for the thinking person but to follow the path from the darkness of illusion towards the light of truth, even if not very much can be hoped for in the way of light or truth. The mechanical perfection of the modern world, where many problems of living appear to have been solved by technology, is accompanied by an almost total loss of a sense of reality in the individual. The inner voice of consciousness is passing judgement and finds the world meaningless, but this nihilism is really a paradox. The mind that passes judgement on the meaninglessness of the universe could not do so if it did not have a deep intuition that meaning might exist. The battle with the will to destruction may be seen as lost but it is still a possibility. The self seeks to know and be known, to confide and to communicate. So while modern literature proclaims nihilism it represents a continuous effort at self-revelation and communion.

It is recognised today that perception and reason are always informed by imagination. The world tends to ratify and open up according to the character of the vision directed towards it. It is no longer possible to think about the world as separate from the mind that knows it. There is now a new romanticism in the reconciliation of subject and object – humanity and nature, spirit and matter, conscious and unconscious, intellect and soul. We have been through an era when the human mind abstracted from the whole all purpose and meaning and claimed them for itself, so that the world was projected as a machine. It was psychoanalysis that began to reverse this process and put man back in touch with the deeper levels of the mind.

The idea of an unconscious mind began to take shape soon after Descartes' time. Science began as a movement towards human freedom, but the separation of mental and physical into separate categories gradually became a double bind which in our time has alienated man from nature. Goethe was one of the writers who preceded Freud in locating the origin of poetic inspiration in the unconscious. All the time there has been an alternative view, which never really went away, that the relationship of the human mind to the world is not dualistic but participatory. In this view the mind is the organ of the world's own process of self-revelation. Nature becomes intelligible to itself through the human mind. To quote Goethe, in a prose translation of a sonnet:

> You must, in studying Nature, always consider both each single thing and the whole: nothing is inside and nothing is outside, for what is within is without. Make haste, then, to grasp this holy mystery which is public knowledge. Rejoice in the true illusion, in the serious game: no living thing is a unity, it is always manifold. (Goethe 1964: 273)

When imaginative understanding is absent, life becomes mechanical. For example, a hypothetical patient visits his doctor complaining of a pain. Investigations are carried out to diagnose the probable disorders giving rise to such a pain. If all the tests come back negative the doctor tells the patient there is nothing the matter with him. The patient still has his pain, which is just as real as before. He now has also a sense of shame, being deprived of a reason for his experience of pain. This scenario is still around, but fortunately less often than it used to be. Many manifestations of inner life are dismissed because there is no rational explanation for them. Intuition, thought transference, prophetic dreams and tele-kinesis are part of many people's experience but they have no scientific explanation. Experiments to test the validity of such phenomena often produce negative results, which is not surprising. Methods of investigation which exclude subjectivity are unlikely to find evidence of it. Fortunately there is a growing interest in subjectivity in many sciences, and hard evidence is accumulating.

The wisdom of previous societies, where it was understood that everything is connected by its meaning, has largely been lost. Only a minority of people understand that science is only one way of looking at the world. Meanwhile momentous changes have been occurring within science itself. Freud's view of mental energy was an extension of the laws of Newtonian physics, which at the time seemed rock-like in their unchangeability. These laws of cause and effect still hold good for practical purposes, but they now have limits. In astronomy and in particle physics the situation is quite different. Einstein's theory of relativity contradicts Newton's notion of time, and quantum physics reveals that at the level of subatomic particles uncertainty and ambiguity prevail. The incompatibility of these two theories means that we are now even farther away from the mechanical universe which Freud inhabited.

Freud presented his structural theory of ego id and superego as a scientific hypothesis. The self is a concept of a different order, in that it refers to subjective experience. Goethe wrote that he did not feel he had dealt with an experience until he had discharged it in creative activity. Freud seems to have used this as a model when he first constructed his theory of mental energy. As a neurologist he was familiar with the spinal reflex arc, in which a sensory input produces a motor discharge (Freud and Breuer 1893). It was natural for him to think of psychic energy being discharged in the same way. Unfortunately this did not work, and it is such mechanical aspects of psychoanalytic theory which now seem the most obsolete.

Self-exploration is necessary in order to develop an identity. We do not automatically know who we are. We like to think of ourselves as rational beings whose lives are governed by the laws of cause and effect. Such beliefs continue despite the obvious fact that the number of variables in any situation makes prediction very unreliable. At the same time, if we do meet someone who behaves in a totally logical manner we soon come to feel that there is something wrong with him. There is more to being human than being rational. Freud was unable to formulate a satisfactory theory of affects because emotions are involved with value judgements, and so are incompatible with his scientific intentions. By excluding the subjective it became impossible to think about the self in moral terms. The essence of human subjectivity is that the self exists in moral space.

People understand intuitively that to ask questions about who a person is, as if it is a scientific experiment, is to miss the point. A self can only exist among other selves. The isolated person does not achieve proper selfhood. One cannot make sense of who a person is without taking other people into account. As a result of Freud's classification the ego is predominant in people's minds when they think about the self and psychoanalytic theory.

There is far more to the self than the ego, and both id and superego involve moral values. Freud's supposedly value-free notion of psychoanalytic theory implies that every child passes through the stages of development and arrives at adulthood. We all know this does not happen; the adult self reflects events at all stages of a person's development. There is a profound difference in quality between infantile sexuality and adult genitality. Growing up involves the partial renunciation of childhood fantasies through reality testing. The child's love for his parents places him centre-stage. The child can only think of his parents needs in terms of his own wishes and knowledge. Infantile omnipotence is almost total subjectivity; the child experiences events with himself as central. If the child's parents separate, he thinks it is his fault because the child cannot think any other way. The child has no choice about his feelings, but his guilt represents a moral choice.

Freud's stage of adult genitality does not mean biological maturity, but the capacity to engage responsibly with a partner experienced as an other, separate and ultimately unknowable. Freud described the process of sublimation whereby immediate gratification is sacrificed in the pursuit of a longer-term aim. The same process is expressed in Goethe's love poems in terms of renunciation. In so far as we keep our infantile omnipotence or narcissism as adults we still think egocentrically, and fail to see and value other people as separate. In clinical practice it is these partial failures of maturation which are revealed. The transference consists of the patient re-experiencing his original fantasies and desires in the relationship to the analyst. The shift from the state of infantile omnipotence to awareness of others involves the development of the capacity to symbolise, which is essential in the development of the self.

We cannot think about the true self without Winnicott's theory of the false self. Every child develops defences against pain and impingement which become the basis of character formation. Clinically, Winnicott's great contribution is that he described the false self as a caretaker self which only allows the true self to emerge when it is safe to do so. This apparently simple statement implies very complex processes, both conscious and unconscious. We can ask, Who is the person who decides that it is safe to be oneself in a particular situation? We soon find that traditional scientific or logical analysis fails to describe the experience that we have.

The false self with which we meet other people is often a compliant self. Winnicott wrote about the spontaneous gesture the baby makes towards the mother, and the need for that gesture to be met by an answering response. If the gesture is not met, the child becomes compliant to the mother's behaviour and some degree of spontaneity is lost. In psychoanalysis the dialogue between therapist and patient allows learned patterns of compliant behaviour to be relived. When the patient comes to understand how the past is being repeated, more straightforward patterns based on self-knowledge begin to replace the symptom-producing compliant ones. It can happen that analyst and patient are surprised by what emerges, but in the long run the discoveries of therapy are rediscoveries of what was once known but had been forgotten or denied.

The basic questions we all need to ask about the meaning of life are not answered by science. The more we learn about the world, the more we realise how little we know. Freud wrote in 'The Interpretation of Dreams':

The unconscious is the true psychical reality; in its innermost nature it is as much unknown to us as the reality of the external world, and it is as incompletely presented by the data of consciousness as is the external world by the communications of our sense organs. (Freud, 1900: 613)

He goes on to refer to Goethe's account of how his new creations came to him without premeditation and almost ready made.

This passage allows us to see Goethe as Freud's inspiration for his description of primary process. Freud's idea of psychic reality has been handed down to us in a restricted version, because of the strong bias towards rationality. Reading Freud with Goethe in mind restores the balance and significance of Freud's extraordinary vision, which may well have been a Goethean science of the mind. Goethe wrote:

> Since it is not possible in either knowledge or reflection to construct a whole, we must necessarily think of science as an art if we expect any kind of wholeness from it ... none of the human faculties should therefore be excluded from scientific activity. The dark depths of prescience, a sure intuition of the present, mathematical profundity, physical accuracy, the heights of reason, an acute understanding, a versatile and ardent imagination, a loving delight in the world of the senses – they are all essential for a lively and productive apprehension of the moment. (Nisbet, 1972: 68–9)

I think Freud would have accepted this as a description of his own ideals.

Our understanding of psychoanalysis is being transformed by the breaking down of the rigid categories of science. There is an explosion of new knowledge which cuts across boundaries between disciplines. A great deal is known about the functions of various parts of the brain, for example, but this tells us the how and not the why of the mind. Now that science has become concerned with subjectivity and with consciousness itself, we can look forward to a new appreciation of the wholeness of the human mind. And this is where Goethe comes in. He was one of the last generation to inherit a world filled with meaning, to understand the connectedness of humankind and nature, and to participate fully. My aim is to show that through the passage of time and changing world views, psychoanalysis can be seen as reaffirming what has been lost. Primary process, the life force, continually renews itself.

Goethe thought his scientific investigations were more important than his poetry. He saw that the scientific method which came into full flower in his lifetime was not the only possible one; it was inadequate for dealing with the phenomena of life and growth because the process of becoming eludes the categories of cause and effect. Science is now catching up with him. I will quote the biologist Mae-Wan Ho:

> The essence of organic wholeness is that it is distributed through-out its constituent parts so that local and global, part and whole are completely indistinguishable. The organism's activities are fully coordinated in a continuum from the molecular to the macro-scopic. There is something very special about the wholeness of organisms that is only captured by quantum coherence. An intuitive appreciation of quantum coherence is to think of the I that each of us experiences as our own being. We know that our body is a multiplicity of organs and tissues, consisting of many billions of cells and astronomical numbers of molecules, all capable of working autonomously and yet somehow cohering into the singular being of our private experience. That is just the stuff of quantum coherence. (Ho 1996: 241)

It is also just the stuff of Goethe's perception of nature, and it could also be an account of Freud's concept of primary process. Goethe's theory of metamorphosis was that organisms must continually change in order to be themselves. This view is now current again; organising principles are recognised in all levels of structure, including the simplest, and within individual cells. The concept of information has replaced mass and energy as the key to understanding life.

Consciousness can be seen as a sense organ for the percep-tion of inner mental activity. The unconscious mind is there-fore similar in kind to all the other natural processes of which we have knowledge. The distinction between mind and body is a distinction between different perceptual modalities. The brain does not exist separately from being experienced. The essence of human thought is the interconnectedness of all things once the duality of alienation has been overcome through self-knowledge.

If there is a unifying self, surely it is that self which creates our dreams. A century on we can see, much better than Freud could, that there is a limit to a rational understanding of dreams. It is the essential creativity and unpredictability of dreams which lie at the heart of psychoanalysis. Primary process thinking has its own logic, which forms the basis of the personality. Freud understood how the events of the day were interwoven with past memories in the formation of dream images. He described how the process of condensation and the elimination of time and contradiction produced the dream thoughts. However, it is no longer possible to hold his other view, that this subtle process has as its aim the discharge of repressed wishes. The only sensible view is that waking and dreaming consciousness are complementary forms of mental activity. Dreaming is an ancient function which we share with animals. It is likely that it plays a role in the survival of the species. The aim of psychoanalysis is the recovery of a sense of belonging in the world through getting in touch with aspects of the self that were disowned in childhood. Paying attention to our dreams is one way of reversing the splitting processes that fragment society. In this way psychoanalysis connects us with the pre-enlightenment state of participation.

In conclusion, the essentials of psychoanalysis are reaffirmed by these new developments in science. Analysts have been subtly influenced by the changes in the world over the decades so that modern practice bears little relationship to the supposedly value-free psychoanalysis that Freud first conceived. Repression and disguise are not required to the extent they were in Freud's Vienna. The changes in society are reflected in patients' dreams, which always have a cultural dimension. The growth in self-awareness that the Freudian revolution produced has resulted in much greater openness to self-understanding. Psychoanalysis can offer a more positive outlook than the self-referential post-modern view of the world. The biological roots of psychoanalysis contradict the current nihilism. If mind and nature are no longer separated, we can return to our roots in dreaming to find answers to our questions about how to live.

References

Arieti, S. (1976) *Creativity: The Magic Synthesis.* New York: Basic Books.

Bakan, D. (1966) *The Duality of Human Existence.* Chicago: Rand McNally.

Barfield, O. (1988) *Saving the Appearances.* Middletown: Wesleyan University Press.

Bateson, G. (1973) *Steps to an Ecology of Mind.* London: Paladin.

Bateson, G. (1979) *Mind and Nature: A Necessary Unity.* New York: Wildwood House; London: Fontana Paperbacks, 1980.

Bettelheim, B. (1983) *Freud and Man's Soul.* London: Chatto and Windus.

Bohm, D. (1980) *Wholeness and the Implicate Order.* London: Routledge and Kegan Paul; Ark paperbacks 1983.

Bollas, C. (1987) *The Shadow of the Object.* London: Free Association Books.

Bollas, C. (1989) *Forces of Destiny.* London: Free Association Books.

Brierley, M. (1932) 'Some problems of integration in women'. *Int. J. Psychoanal.* 13: 433–48.

Brierley, M. (1944) 'Psychoanalytic theory', in *Trends in Psychoanalysis.* London: Hogarth Press.

Brierley, M. (1951) *Trends in Psychoanalysis.* London: Hogarth Press.

Burrow, T. (1973) *The Preconscious Foundations of Human Experience.* New York: Basic Books.

Coltart, N. (1985) 'Slouching towards Bethlehem', in G. Kohon, ed. *The British School of Psychoanalysis: the Independent Tradition*, 185–99. London: Free Association Books.

Coltart, N. (1990) 'Attention'. *Brit. J. Psychotherapy*, 7: 64–74.

Coltart, N. (1993) *Slouching towards Bethlehem*. London: Free Association Books.

Cupitt, D. (1980) *Taking Leave of God*. London: SCM Press.

Duncan, D. (1990) 'The Feel of the Session'. *Psychoanalysis and Contemporary Thought*, 13: 3–22.

Freud, S. (1900) 'The Interpretation of Dreams', in J. Strachey, ed., *The Standard Edition of the Complete Psychological Works of Sigmund Freud*, 24 vols. Hogarth, 1953–73, vols 4 and 5.

Freud, S. (1915a) 'The Unconscious', *S.E.* 14.

Freud, S. (1915b) *A Phylogenetic Fantasy*. E. Grubrich-Simitis, ed. Cambridge, Mass: Harvard University Press, 1987.

Freud, S. (1927) 'The Future of an Illusion'. *S.E.* 21, 5–56.

Freud, S. (1933) 'Why War?' *S.E.* 22, 197–215.

Freud, S. and Breuer, J. (1893) 'Studies in Hysteria' *S.E.* 2.

Galatzer-Levy, R. (1978) 'Qualitative change from quantitative change'. *J. Am. Psychoanal. Assoc.* 26: 921–35.

Gillespie, W.H. (1969) 'Concepts of Vaginal Orgasm'. *Int. J. Psychoanal.* 50: 495–7.

Gillespie, W.H. (1975) 'Woman and her Discontents'. *Int. Rev. Psychoanal.* 2: 1–10.

Gleick, J. (1987) *Chaos*. London: Heinemann and Cardinal paperbacks.

Goethe, J.W. (1964) *Selected Verse*. Edited and with prose translations by D. Luke. London: Penguin Classics.

Goodwin, B. (1994) *How the Leopard Changed its Spots*. London: Weidenfeld and Nicholson; Phoenix Giant 1995.

Ho, M.-W. (1996) The Biology of Free Will. *Journal of Consciousness Studies*, 3(3): 231–45.

Hobsbawm, E. (1994) *The Age of Extremes*. London: Viking Penguin.

Home, J. (1966) 'The Concept of Mind'. *Int. J. Psychoanal.* 47: 43–9.

Jantsch, E. (1980) *The Self-organising Universe*. Oxford: Pergamon.

Jung, C.G. (1927) 'The structure of the psyche'. *Collected Works* VIII. Reprinted in A. Storr, ed. *Jung: Selected writings*. Fontana Pocket Readers, 1983, 66–8.

Jung, C.G. and Pauli, W. (1955) 'On the nature of the psyche'.

C. W. VIII. Reprinted in A. Storr, ed. *Jung: Selected writings.* Fontana Pocket Readers, 1983, 336–9.

Kuhn, T. (1962) *The Structure of Scientific Revolutions.* Chicago: Chicago University Press.

Lamarck, J-B. (1809) *Zoological Philosophy,* trans by H. Elliott. New York and London: Hafner Press.

Langer, S. (1942) *Philosophy in a New Key.* London: Oxford University Press. Reprinted in Harvard paperbacks, 1978.

Lovejoy, A.O. (1936) *The Great Chain of Being.* Cambridge, Mass: Harvard University Press. Reprinted in paperback.

Lovelock, J. (1982) *Gaia.* Oxford: Oxford University Press.

Mahlberg, A. (1987) 'Evidence of Collective memory; a test of Sheldrake's theory'. *Journal of Analytical Psychol.* 32(1): 23–34.

Matte Blanco, I. (1975) *The Unconscious as Infinite Sets.* London: Duckworth.

Milner, M. (1952) 'Aspects of Symbolism in the Comprehension of the not-self'. *Int. J. Psychoanal.* 33: 181–95.

Modell, A. (1981) 'Does metapsychology still exist?' *Int. J. Psychoanal.* 62: 391–402.

Nisbet, H.B. (1972) *Goethe and the Scientific Tradition.* London: Institute of Germanic Studies.

Noll, R. (1994) *The Jung Cult.* Princeton: Princeton University Press.

Ornston, D. (1982) 'Strachey's Influence: A preliminary report'. *Int. J. Psychoanal.* 63: 409–26.

Parsons, M. (1984) 'Psychoanalysis as vocation and martial art'. *Int. Rev. Psychoanal.* 11: 453–62.

Parsons, M. (1990) 'Marion Milner's "Answering activity" and the question of psychoanalytic creativity'. *Int. Rev. Psychoanal.* 17: 413–24.

Pauli, W. (1955) 'The influence of archetypal ideas on the scientific theories of Kepler', in C.G. Jung and W. Pauli, *The Interplay of Nature and the Psyche,* New York: Bollingen, 1963.

Payne, S.M. (1935) 'A concept of femininity'. *Brit. J. Med. Psychol.* 15: 18–33.

Peat, F.D. (1988) *Synchronicities.* New York: Bantam.

Piaget, J. (1947) *The Psychology of Intelligence.* London: Routledge & Kegan Paul.

Polanyi, M. (1958) *Personal Knowledge.* London: Routledge and Kegan Paul.

Pribram, K. (1976) 'Transcendentalism and the logical paradox', in G.C. Globus et al; eds., *Consciousness and the Brain.* New York: Plenum Press.

Pribram, K. (1989) 'Psychoanalysis and the natural sciences', in J. Sandler, ed. *Dimensions of Psychoanalysis.* London: Karnac.

Rayner, E. (1981) 'Infinite experiences, affects and the characteristics of the unconscious'. *Int. J. Psychoanal.* 62: 403–12.

Reed, T.J. (1984) *Goethe.* Past Masters series. Oxford: Oxford University Press.

Riviere, J. (1934) 'Review of Freud's "New introductory lectures"'. *Int. J. Psychoanal.* 15: 329–39.

Rycroft, C. (1956) 'The nature of the analyst's communication to the patient'. *Int. J. Psychoanal.* 37: 469–72. Reprinted in Rycroft (1968b).

Rycroft, C. (1962) 'Beyond the reality principle'. *Int. J. Psychoanal.* 43: 388–94.

Rycroft, C. (1968a) *A Critical Dictionary of Psychoanalysis.* London: Nelson. 1995 second edn revised, London: Penguin.

Rycroft, C. (1968b) *Imagination and Reality.* London: Hogarth Press.

Rycroft, C. (1979) *The Innocence of Dreams.* London: Hogarth Press.

Rycroft, C. (1985) 'Psychoanalysis and the literary imagination', in *Psychoanalysis and Beyond.* London: Chatto Tigerstripe.

Sharpe, E.F. (1935) 'Similar and divergent unconscious determinants underlying the sublimations of pure art and pure science'. *Int. J. Psychoanal.* 16: 186–202.

Sheldrake, A.R. (1981) *A New Science of Life: The Hypothesis of Formative Causation.* London: Blond & Briggs. Second edn 1985.

Spruiell, V. (1993) 'Deterministic Chaos and the Sciences of Complexity: Psychoanalysis in the Midst of a General Scientific Revolution'. *J. Am. Psychoanal. Assoc.* 41: 3–44.

Stern, D. (1985) *The Interpersonal World of the Infant.* New York: Basic Books.

Storr, A. (1985) 'Psychoanalysis and Creativity', in P. Horden, ed. *Psychoanalysis and the Humanities.* London: Duckworth. Reprinted in *Churchill's Black Dog.* London: Collins, 1985.

Storr, A. (1987) 'Jung's conception of personality', in A. Peacocke and G. Gillett, eds *Persons and Personality.* Oxford: Blackwell.

Thom, R. (1978) *Structural stability and Morphogenesis.* Reading, Mass: Addison Wesley.

Trevarthen, C. (1994) 'Brain Development, Infant Communication and Empathy Disorders'. *Development and Psychopathology,* 1994, 6(4): 597–633.

Ullman, M. (1993) 'Dreams, the Dreamer and Society' in G. Delaney (ed.) *New Directions in Dream Interpretation.* New York: State University of New York Press.

Ullman, M., Krippner, S. and Vaughan, A. (1973) *Dream Telepathy.* New York: Macmillan.

Ullman, M. and Zimmerman, N. (1979) *Working with Dreams.* New York: Jeremy P. Tarcher/Perigee.

Waddington, C.H. (1957) *The Strategy of the Genes.* London: Allen and Unwin.

Wallace, A.R. (1911) *The World of Life: A Manifestation of Creative Power, Directive Mind and Ultimate Purpose.* London: Chapman Hall.

Whitehead, A.N. (1925) *Science and the Modern World.* New York: Macmillan.

Winnicott, D.W. (1965) 'Ego Distortion in Terms of True and False Self' in *The Maturational Process and the Facilitating Environment.* London: Hogarth Press.

Winnicott, D.W. (1971a) 'Creativity and its origins'. in *Playing and Reality.* London: Tavistock.

Winnicott, D.W. (1971b) 'Transitional Objects and transitional phenomena', in *Playing and Reality.* London: Tavistock.

Yankelovich, D. and Barrett, W. (1970) *Ego and Instinct.* New York: Random House.

Zeeman, C. (1977) *Catastrophe Theory.* New York: Addison Wesley.

Zinkin, L. (1984) 'The hologram as a model for analytical psychology'. *J. Analytical Psychol.* 32: 1–21.

Index

Index compiled by
Auriol Griffith-Jones